SpringerBriefs in Well-Being and Quality of Life Research

W0079258

More information about this series at http://www.springer.com/series/10150

Valerie Michaelson · Nathan King
William Pickett

Holistic Health in Children: Conceptualization, Assessment and Potential

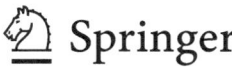 Springer

Valerie Michaelson
Department of Public Health Sciences and
  School of Religion
Queen's University
Kingston, ON
Canada

William Pickett
Department of Public Health Sciences
Queen's University
Kingston, ON
Canada

Nathan King
Department of Public Health Sciences
Queen's University
Kingston, ON
Canada

ISSN 2211-7644   ISSN 2211-7652   (electronic)
SpringerBriefs in Well-Being and Quality of Life Research
ISBN 978-3-319-64830-9   ISBN 978-3-319-64831-6   (eBook)
DOI 10.1007/978-3-319-64831-6

Library of Congress Control Number: 2017947485

Printed on acid-free paper

This Springer imprint is published by Springer Nature
The registered company is Springer International Publishing AG
The registered company address is: Gewerbestrasse 11, 6330 Cham, Switzerland

Acknowledgements

We would first like to thank the many young people who participated in the qualitative studies that are described in this small book. While we have a commitment to protecting your identity, we want to recognize how thoughtful your ideas were, and how much we enjoyed talking to each and every one of you! We would also like to thank the terrific artists who helped to illustrate this book: Lily, Catia, Isabel and Isobel.

Dr. Colleen Davison conceived and led the initial Childhealth 2.0 Canadian Institutes of Health Research project on which this study was based, and we thank her for her vision and support. We also thank the research assistants who were involved in various phases of this project: Sophie Moore, Hannah Ascough and Emma Lockhart, and Dr. Jennifer Taylor. Eleanor Vandermeer assisted with the analysis reported in Chap. 2, and parts of that analysis were previously published in the International Journal of Qualitative Studies on Health and Well-being (volume 11, 2016) under the title "A mixed methods study of Canadian adolescents' perceptions of health". We acknowledge our co-authors for that manuscript, Colleen Davison, Eleanor Vandermeer and Brian Taylor. We are also grateful to Mr. David Hannah, educational consultant at Bayridge Secondary School in Kingston, Dr. Nancy Dalgarno, Education Researcher and Consultant, Office of Health Sciences Education/Department of Family Medicine-Centre for Studies in Primary Care, Faculty of Health Sciences, Queen's University and Dr. Susan Phillips, Clinical Practitioner and Queen's University Department of Family Medicine, who provided important insights into Chap. 5. Our editor Bren Melles and graphic artist Lesley Lorimer made important contributions to the final document.

The Public Health Agency of Canada and Health Canada funded Cycle 7 of the Health Behaviour in School-aged Children (HBSC) study in Canada. International Coordinator of the 2014 HBSC survey was Dr. Candace Currie, University of St. Andrews, Scotland. The international databank manager was Dr. Oddrun Samdal, University of Bergen, Norway. The Canadian Principal Investigators of the 2014 HBSC study were Drs. John Freeman and William Pickett, Queen's University; its National Coordinator was Matthew King. We also thank the

Pan-Canadian Joint Consortium for School Health (JCSH; Executive Director, Katherine Kelly) for its counsel with respect to the 2014 HBSC survey design and administration in Canada. Additional support for this analysis included an operating grant from the Canadian Institutes of Health Research (CIHR Grant FRN 130379).

The funders had no role in study design, data collection and analysis, decision to publish, or preparation of this book.

Contents

Chapter 1
Introduction to Holism

> *When we try to pick out anything by itself we find it hitched to everything else in the Universe.*
>
> —John Muir

> *I think it means that it is ... beneficial to look at health all at once ... like in school ... if we take health we would probably do a couple of classes on nutrition and a couple on safety and then some on exercise and that kind of thing. But we never really look at everything all at once ....*
>
> —Focus group participant

Abstract In this first chapter of this small book, we introduce the theory of holism in simple terms. We revisit its historic roots, including insights from Indigenous approaches to health and wellness, and then we discuss the more recent re-emergence of holism in ideas and debates in the field of health promotion, including those that involve children. This theoretical framework lays the foundation for the main purpose of this book, which is very simple and practical: to apply basic principles of holism to many aspects of the health of children.

Keywords Holism · Indigenous · Children · Child health · Reductionism

What makes a child healthy? Is it eating a nutritious diet, getting the right amount of physical activity, or living smoke free? Is a child's health grounded in a supportive family life or based on access to quality health services? Or is it even broader than that, including cultural values, equality and dignity?

It seems obvious that the health of children does not depend on just one thing. But sometimes when we think about health, we break it down into smaller and smaller pieces with the idea that the best way to understand something is to isolate and analyze the smallest and simplest parts (Ahn, Tewari, Poon, & Phillips, 2006; Atun, 2012; Swanson et al. 2012). There is certainly value in this approach. But might there be another way to think about child health that looks not at the pieces, but at the whole? In other words, is there value in an approach to child health that is holistic?

© The Author(s) 2018
V. Michaelson et al., *Holistic Health in Children: Conceptualization, Assessment and Potential*, SpringerBriefs in Well-Being and Quality of Life Research, DOI 10.1007/978-3-319-64831-6_1

A simple example illustrates what we mean by holistic: a birthday cake. Each component that goes into that cake—its basic ingredients of butter and sugar, flour, eggs, baking soda and milk, and its equally important elements of care and skill in the baker—have their own unique properties. But when these ingredients are combined in a particular way, the parts combine to create something new altogether. When a child looks at the cake, she doesn't think "butter, sugar, flour, eggs and candles". For this child, the whole is much more than the sum of all the parts. It includes not only a delicious cake, but something that cannot be measured in terms of human relationships, care and value. This is holism.

While holism is compelling as a theory, we recognize that our ability to actually apply it to the diverse field of adolescent health is challenging. In Chaps. 2 and 3, we use qualitative methods to help us understand how holistic concepts of health can be meaningfully applied to child populations. In Chap. 4, we explore some novel analytic methods that have been used to model health and its determinants holistically, and discuss quantitative approaches to the creation of holistic health indicators. Inspired by analytic methods from UNICEF (Adamson, 2010), we apply these to the development of new composite measures of adolescent health and its contextual/individual determinants. We also outline the importance of such composite measures as applied to the assessment of both potential causes, and the promotion of, health within adolescent populations. In the final chapter, we integrate our findings and consider application for the health of children. Brief methods for each of these studies are included in Chaps. 2 through 4, and full methods are found in Appendices A, B and C.

Our hope is that through this book, we can apply holistic thinking and models to issues of health, particularly in children. This kind of thinking has the potential to provide new insights that can inform research and health education/promotion strategies. Indeed, in order to understand a child, we must look at the child as a whole person within a context. And further, like the metaphorical birthday cake, the way the parts all come together and interact results in something much more profound than the flour, sugar, butter and eggs.

Defining Holistic Child Health

Thinking about health holistically is not an original idea. From ancient texts to high-level contemporary research journals, holistic ideas about health have been considered for millennia. The word "health" itself provides an etymological clue as to the importance of the close relationship between holism and health. The English word *health* was derived from the Old English word *haelp* (wholeness, a being whole, sound or well) and the Old Norse *helge* (holy or sacred). The word is connected to the root *kailo* (whole), then *haelan* (to make whole). The same root is connected to the Greek word *holos* (whole) and to the modern English word "holistic" (Online Etymology Dictionary, 2017). Etymologically, one could thus argue that the concepts of "health", "wholeness" and "holism" at a minimum overlap, and almost certainly are interconnected.

Even a cursory review of literature related to holism and health demonstrates a large variety of understanding of the concept of holism as it relates to health. The word holistic is used to describe complementary or alternative approaches to medicine, health and healing, but is also found in more mainstream journals such as the *British Medical Journal*, the *British Journal of Nursing, the Lancet* and *Pediatrics*. By definition, this theory suggests that *organic or unified 'wholes' have value and qualities which are inherently different from, and cannot be reduced to, the sum of their individual parts* (Christakis, 2012; Michaelson, Pickett, King, & Davison, 2016).

The Oxford Living Dictionary (English Oxford Living Dictionary, 2016), defines holism in two ways:

First, in terms of philosophy, holism is "[t]he theory that parts of a whole are in intimate interconnection, such that they cannot be understood without reference to the whole, which is thus regarded as greater than the sum of its parts...." And second, in terms of medicine, holism is defined as "[t]he treating of the whole person, taking into account mental and social factors, rather than just the symptoms of a disease" (English Oxford Living Dictionary, 2016).

We draw from both of these definitions, and also from the ideas of Stempsey (2001, p. 202) and Phillips (1976) to construct a framework to guide our work. We thus understand something that is holistic to have two distinct properties. First, the whole is more than the sum of the parts, and there is an emergent property in the whole that is not reflected by the component parts. And second, the parts are interconnected, and gain new meaning in connection to each other and to the whole. We will revisit this basic framework throughout this book.

Holism and Health: A Historical Overview

As we have related, the theory of holism is an ancient concept. Written records from Ancient Greek civilizations reveal connections between the concept of holism and the field of health. For example, as early as the 4th century BCE, Plato, in his play Charmides, gives Socrates the line "the part can never be well unless the whole is well" as he discusses a cure for Charmides' headache (Plato, 380 BCE). In Stempsey's analysis of Plato, he observes that for Plato, health is more than a healthy body. It is an integration of body and soul; "it is a vision of the good life itself." (Stempsey, 2001, p. 209).

Many ancient and contemporary Indigenous approaches to health, wellness and associated care are also holistic, and take a broad ecological approach to health. They consider the balance not only of the spiritual, emotional, physical and intellectual dimensions of a person acting as an individual, but also as a member of a family, community and nation in a variety of cultural, social, economic and political environments. (Graham & Leeseberg-Stamler, 2010; Griffiths, 1998; Tagalik, 2010; Wollumbin, 2012). Integral to Indigenous health is regaining balance, which can be achieved by building relationships with others, taking care of oneself and following a cultural path (Hunter, Logan, Goulet, & Barton, 2006). A strong illustration of this concept of balance is found in the Medicine Wheel, "one of the basic symbols of the world view of First Nations" (Svenson & Lafontaine, 1999). Its underlying philosophy suggests that health is best viewed as an interconnected phenomenon that cannot be understood apart from a person's environmental context (Svenson & Lafontaine, 1999). Further, it emphasizes the relatedness of the physical, mental, emotional, and spiritual dimensions of being, and also their application to healing oneself and one's relationships (Graham & Leeseberg-Stamler, 2010; NCCAH, 2013). Indigenous approaches are increasingly acknowledged as complementary to many views of modern medicine. Indeed, in recognition of the deep relevance of Indigenous concepts of health and healing, the Indigenous Physicians Association of Canada (IPAC) and the Association of Faculties of Medicine of Canada (AFMC) created a set of competency standards for medical students working with First Nations, Inuit, and Métis patients (Indigenous Physicians Association of Canada & The Association of Faculties of Medicine of Canada (IPAC & AFMC), 2009).

Canadian contemporary Indigenous cultures are not alone in connecting holism and health. In both ancient and modern Judaism, for example, the Hebrew word *shalom*, exchanged at meeting and/or parting, is used to mean the fullness—or wholeness—of what health can be—i.e., the idea of "completeness, soundness, well-being, wholeness, peace, and health" (Strong, 2005). As such, it includes the person, their place in this world, and the matrix of relationships that shape their life. Shalom relates to a dynamic sense of a person flourishing in the context of healthy relationships, and also bringing healing, reconciliation, and peace into the troubled and broken relationships around them. Shalom deepens our understanding of the fullness—or wholeness—of what health can be, and brings with it a picture of health in its broadest, most integrative sense.

The traditional Southern African philosophy of Ubuntu, too, offers a holistic understanding of ourselves at a societal level, in relation to the world and people around us (Edwards, Makunga, Ngcobo, & Dhlomo, 2012). Not unlike Shalom, the central concepts of Ubuntu are about human interdependence and relatedness. It is the recognition that we are all connected, and that the flourishing of one person relates to the flourishing of all. Ubuntu has been used as the foundation of programs in children's palliative care (Marston, 2015), nursing (Downing & Hastings-Tolsma, 2016; Mulaudzi, Libster, & Phiri, 2009) and to address the HIV/AIDS crisis in parts of Africa (Bessler, 2008). This philosophy pushes our ideas of holistic health beyond scientifically measureable constructs (such as height, weight, social capital and relative affluence) to attributes of kindness, vulnerability and belonging.

Holism in the 20th Century

The actual term "holism" was proposed in 1926 by South African Jan Smuts. In his book *Holism and Evolution*, Smuts wrote about how he was captivated with the idea that "the particular only acquired meaning as part of the greater whole" (1926, p. 14). Smuts argued that holism is the idea that natural systems (e.g., physical, biological, or social) and their properties should be viewed not as a collection of parts, but as integrated wholes.[1]

The ideas that Smuts articulated early in the 20th century took hold in modern science, and certainly, this holistic science that arose in the 1920s was both "real" science *and* a "profoundly cultural discourse" (Harrington, 1996, p. 208). This may well—at least in part—explain why over the last century Smuts' initial ideas have evolved and are recognizable in fields as diverse as ecology, agriculture, psychiatry, biology, education and theology. Increasingly, the relationship between scientific discovery and human meaning was being held together by holistic approaches in all kinds of disciplines. Along with this, it was being recognized that complex problems needed holistic approaches and solutions, ones that drew from a variety of disciplines, lenses and views.

While definitions and applications of the theory of holism have evolved, the basic ideas can still be traced back to Smuts. The multi-disciplinary and holistic discussion that arose from his work became a challenge to modernity's attempts to "strip the world of meaning" by its attempts to cut it up into smaller and smaller pieces in our efforts to gain understanding (Zelko, 2012, p. 17). It is perhaps no surprise then, that in 1936, Albert Einstein wrote that along with relativity, holism would be one of the two mental constructs that would direct human thinking in the next millennium (Einstein, 1936). Over the last century, the concept of holism has been applied in fields as diverse as biology (Isberg & Falkow, 1985; Kitano, 2002), ecology (Kitching, 1983; Odum, 1994), physics (Böhm & Hiley, 1993), philosophy (Katinić, 2013), anthropology (Harkin, 2010) and economics (Fullerton, 2015).

For our purposes, we are most interested in how holistic thinking has been applied in disciplines that focus on the health and well-being of humans. Fast-forward 75 years from Einstein, and we see that modern health promotion efforts have

---

[1]Smuts makes a clear distinction between mechanical systems (which are, to Smuts, not holistic because the parts "retain their own distinctive properties regardless of whether they are integrated in the machine or not" (1926/1966, p. 672)) and living systems. A living organism or ecological system is much different, because the whole is "*more* than the sum of its parts" (Smuts, 1926/1966, p. 102). Whereas both living organisms and machines are systems that contain interacting parts, "the nature of the relation between these parts and the system as a whole is very different" (Lundh, 2015, p. 187). The parts of the machine retain their own discrete properties regardless of whether or how they are integrated into the larger machine. The parts of a living organism, however, develop their respective identities out of their relationship to the whole. In other words, the parts cannot exist without their relationship to the whole (Smuts 1926/1966).

adopted holism, including as a foundation for many contemporary World Health Organization approaches to health promotion and policy. These are old—even ancient—ideas, which have found many applications to contemporary society.

Holism and Reductionism: Complementary Approaches to Health

Holism has not always been a popular theory. Looking back to the 17th century, French philosopher René Descartes argued that in order to understand a complex phenomena, one needs to break it down and look at or analyze the smallest and simplest components or parts, in isolation from the whole (Descartes, 1998). This is the basis of the concept of "reductionism". The last several centuries have been largely dominated by various Cartesian approaches to science, which have encouraged breaking matter and bodies down into smaller and smaller bits in the pursuit of understanding.

There is obvious value in reductionist theories and approaches that focus on understanding the individual components and mechanisms that constitute systems. Specific focus on the muscular system, brain development or oral care all have value, as does focus on understanding the importance of individual diseases and their physical and social mechanisms (for example, environmental and genetic determinants of cancer, and what happens at the cellular level for a tumour to develop). This type of understanding is essential for prevention and treatment initiatives. And further, few would argue that understanding the intricacies of the heart, brain or circulatory system are not fundamentally important to helping children to have the best possible health outcomes. Cartesian approaches have hugely advanced our ability to treat the body, and such advances have shown the positive side of reductionist thinking.

But there was also something dubious in this way of thinking. Because of reductionist thinking, entire clinical disciplines became separated from each other, each based on different views of disease and associated pathologies. For example, the International Classification of Diseases, now in its 10th revision, still excludes psychiatric diseases and disorders from its core content (WHO, 1992). And quite frankly, virtually all of the existing classification systems and associated thinking consider disease, organic or psychological, to be something that is best viewed using a compartmentalized lens, including the idea that mental illness is fundamentally separate from illness of the body. The theory of holism suggests that on its own, this type of understanding is incomplete. As Kendell writes, "In reality, neither minds nor bodies develop illnesses. Only people (or, in a wider context, organisms) do so, and when they do, both mind and body, psyche and soma, are usually involved" (2001, p. 491).

A thoughtful theory of holism does not pit holism against reductionism, and does not propose looking only at things in their entirety without any concern for their constituent parts. On the contrary, holistic thinking is complementary to reductionist thinking about health, and incorporates the valid aspects of reductionism while also paying attention to the whole (Járos, 2002).

Contemporary Applications of the Theory of Holism to Health

There are a large variety of ways that holism has been used in contemporary approaches to health. We are going to limit our discussion to four areas: health education, health promotion, health policy, and health research. Our goal is not to provide an exhaustive survey, but rather, to provide a glimpse into the myriad of ways that holistic thinking is already being applied in many health contexts.

Health Education

One way that holistic thinking has been applied is to inform health education. For example, the Ontario health and physical education curriculum for 2015 recognizes health as a "holistic phenomenon" (Ontario Ministry of Education, 2015, p. 34), and encourages students to make connections between different aspects of their health, including physical, mental, spiritual, social and emotional domains. Students also learn about the connections between healthy choices, active living, and chronic disease prevention (p. 34) with the goal that their learning in health education forms an integrated whole that connects to their everyday lives. While individual aspects of health are considered in detail, the overall curriculum encourages students to understand connections between the various component parts.

The Pan-Canadian Joint Consortium for School Health (2017, established in 2005), was developed to forge links between education and health, and offers another example. Recognizing that outcomes in both areas would be better with an integrative and holistic approach, the Consortium champions programs such as Comprehensive School Health (2017), which is an integrative, holistic framework that supports student health in school contexts. In CSH, it is recognized that children can only reach their full potential as learners if their physical, mental, intellectual and emotional needs are met, and their health and education are connected.

Health Promotion

Neither of these two examples of holistic approaches to education emerged from a vacuum, and each was shaped by a dialogue that emerged in the related area of health promotion. One of the early places this was articulated was in the 1986

Ottawa Charter on Health Promotion, which recognizes caring, holism, and ecology as "essential issues in developing strategies for health promotion" (Ottawa Charter, p. 3). The 1997 Jakarta Declaration affirms the Ottawa Charter, and further emphasizes the effectiveness of comprehensive approaches to health promotion over single-track strategies. In both the Ottawa and Jakarta statements, as well as in other World Health Organization documents, an emphasis on the interdependent issues of social justice, human rights, ecology, global sustainability and technology have also arisen (WHO, 1986b, 2009).

A very practical example of the way that these various health promotion documents have informed real practice is found in the WHO's Healthy Settings initiative. Healthy Settings approaches, which are directly rooted in the Ottawa Charter, "involve a holistic and multi-disciplinary method which integrates action across risk factors. The goal is to maximize disease prevention via a "whole system" approach" (WHO, 1986a). This includes key principles such as community participation, partnership, empowerment and equity. Indeed, it pushes boundaries of health to resemble something closer to Ubuntu or Shalom than we might previously have considered. This is just one example of the many ways that holistic thinking is currently considered in health promotion, and is spilling over into real practice.

Health Policy

Holistic and intersectoral approaches to health care and policy are being used in Canada and around the world. Examples of frameworks that draw from holistic approaches include the *Mandala of Health*, which is a Canadian Framework proposed by Hancock and Perkins (1985). This model demonstrates how health is more than individual behaviours, and is "simultaneously influenced by human biology, personal behavior, psychosocial environment, human environment, and natural environment" (p. 27). The Wider Determinants of Health Model (Dahlgren & Whitehead, 1991) is another model that recognizes the myriad of factors that can both hinder and enhance the health status of individuals and populations. And third, using a uniquely First Nations approach, the First Nations Holistic Policy and Planning Model (AFN, 2013) demonstrates how the use of culture can be effective in developing holistic health models. This model holds together essential components of achieving positive health, including justice, economic development, housing and the environment. The Centre for Addiction and Mental Health (CAMH, 2017) in Canada uses what it describes as holistic health to move thinking beyond a biomedical focus and to recognize the synergies between the individual, interpersonal, organizational, community, policy and superstructural levels of a health system (Khenti et al., 2015; Scott & Wilson, 2011; Sweat & Denison, 1995). In each of these examples, the interaction between the various components/spheres/ sectors of health is integral to the efficacy of these models in promoting action on each interconnected aspect of health.

It is worth looking closely at a 2007 policy framework called "People Centred Health Care" (WHO, 2007). This was presented and endorsed by WHO Member States during the fifty-eighth session of the Regional Committee for the Western Pacific that was held in the Republic of Korea. It describes the "complex interplay of physical, social, economic, cultural and environmental factors" (p. 1) and makes a strong call for a more holistic and people-centred approach to health care, one that balances the rights and responsibilities of all stakeholders. In this document too, we find new Ubuntu or Shalom-like language being introduced. Along with quality health care and patient safety, we hear terms like "equity and fairness... human dignity... and the role of families, culture and society" (p. 3). This framework recognizes that expectations and demands around health care delivery are changing, with expectations of a more "humanistic and holistic approach to health care, where the individual who needs care is viewed and respected as a whole person with multidimensional needs" (p. 4). Here again, words such as human rights and dignity, nondiscrimination, participation and empowerment, access and equity, and a partnership of equals are core values for thinking about health (p. 7).

Health Research

The examples so far relate to health promotion, education and policy. One area of particular interest is in finding ways that holistic ideas can be applied to research, and to measurement of health status. A team in Hong Kong has done exciting work in developing and assessing the psychometric properties of a scale designed to measure the holistic care needs of individuals who have been diagnosed with chronic disease (Chan, Wong, Yeung, & Sum, 2016). A systematic literature review led by Dr. de Silva, from the Evidence Centre in the United Kingdom, examines approaches to the measurement of person-centred care. Here she points to what she describes as an increasing number of named and validated tools for measuring person-centred care holistically as well as its specific components (DeSilva, 2014, p. 2). These holistic measures include the Individualised Care Scale (ICS); the Measure of Processes of Care (MOPC); the Person-centred Care Assessment Tool (P-CAT) and the Person-centred Climate Questionnaire (PCCQ). Of the 921 studies included in this review, 55% (503 studies) used holistic measures to focus on person-centred care as a broad holistic concept.

Drawing Boundaries Around Holism

"Everything affects health" writes Freeman (2005, p. 155). For our own work in applying the theory of holism to research with children, we needed to draw some practical boundaries around what we mean by holism, and around how big it can get.

We recognize that thinking about health holistically could easily and quickly get so big that it would lose all practical value when it comes to health promotion and interventions. Indeed, it would not take long for our conversation about the interconnectedness of holistic health to turn to issues of human rights, ecological sustainability, equity, justice and gender relations. These are all issues that cannot be left out of the field of holistic child health, but the danger is that before long, we have left our conversation that is specific to health and are talking about a theory of everything: interesting yes, but not practically useful to our purposes. Here, Freeman's work is helpful. He writes:

> [t]o a certain extent, what is 'holistic' depends upon where you stand....For a cell biologist, holism might mean thinking about the whole liver. In various contexts, it might mean the whole person, the whole community, the whole of society, or the whole planet. Which environmental events you respond to depends on the scale at which you choose to observe ('this person is obese' versus '30% of the US population is obese'). So the largest scale that is relevant to you, that you pay attention to, is probably what you define as holism (Freeman, 2005, p. 155).

One of our challenges is to have a focused conversation about child health, using the theoretical framework of holism. We appreciate that implicit to our ideas is a myriad of synergies, complexities and interactions across all the systems and within all aspects of the individual child that directly and indirectly impact the child. This concept of holistic child health is flexible, and like Freeman, we use it not to talk about a theory of everything, but to look at the largest scale that is relevant to the particular conversation we are having at any given time.

Two Challenges Surrounding Research Related to Holistic Child Health

As we seek to apply the theory of holism to child health, we address two main challenges. The first relates to finding a way to apply our study in a way that is meaningful to adolescent populations. We recognize that today's children conceptualize important components of health in ways that do not fit into historical paradigms. It would be both foolish and futile to find ways to measure health holistically in manners that had no connection to the lives of real children. Our challenge here is to intentionally listen to children, as we are able, in order to understand how they conceptualize health, and further, to understand how health can be discussed and promoted in ways that resonate with their everyday experiences in their own lives.

Our second challenge relates to measurement. In a rapidly evolving world, basic constructs that are thought to constitute health may change, and need to be revisited often. With this in mind, it is not always obvious what the components of health are that most profoundly contribute to a more complete holistic understanding. What was helpful in one time and context may not be as helpful in another. To deepen

this challenge, even if the components that belong in a holistic model were identified, how would one weight such components in models of health, and decide
what thresholds of a specific health attribute, state, behavior or context are meaningful? We address both of these challenges in the next several chapters via a mixed
methods paradigm.

Our Hopes for This Small Book

In this chapter, we have offered a simple overview of the theory of holism, and
provided examples of its utility for the study of health. One fundamental goal of our
efforts to view child health in a holistic manner is to understand what children need
in order to live well and fully in the context of their everyday lives. In the next two
chapters, we address the challenges of measurement and meaningful application of
the concept of holistic health for child and adolescent populations. And, we close
the book with a final chapter that is interpretive and practical.

In the end, by integrating qualitative and quantitative approaches, our hope is to
explore that not only is the whole more than the sum of its parts, but that the whole
potentially contributes to new understanding of the parts. This kind of thinking is
fundamental to holism. It provides opportunities for new insights into health and its
determinants in children and adolescents, including practical recommendations on
implications for both prevention and future research paradigms.

Key Insights from This Chapter

- Something that is holistic has at least two distinct properties

  - Something emerges from the whole that is not reflected by the com-
    ponent parts
  - The parts are interconnected and interdependent

- Holistic thinking is central to many ancient and contemporary views about
  health, including Indigenous health
- Throughout the 20th and 21st centuries, holistic thinking has been applied
  to fields as diverse as ecology, philosophy and economics
- A thoughtful theory of holism as applied to health is not opposed to
  reductionism, but rather incorporates the valid aspects of reductionism
  while also paying attention to the whole
- Challenges to applying holism to child health include:

  - Finding ways to apply holism to health that are meaningful to children
  - Finding useful ways of assessing or measuring health holistically

References

Adamson, P. (2010). *The children left behind: A league table of inequality in child well-being in the world's rich countries. Innocenti Report Card, no. 9.* Florence, Italy: UNICEF Innocenti Research Centre.

AFN. (2013). *First Nations holistic policy and planning a transitional discussion document on the social determinants of health.* Ottawa, Ontario: Assembly of First Nations. Retrieved from http://health.afn.ca/uploads/les/sdoh_afn.pdf.

Ahn, A. C., Tewari, M., Poon, C. S., & Phillips, R. S. (2006). The limits of reductionism in medicine: Could systems biology offer an alternative? *PLoS Med, 3*(6), 709–713.

Atun, R. (2012). Health systems, systems thinking and innovation. *Health Policy and Planning, 27* (suppl 4), iv4–iv8.

Bessler, J. D. (2008). In the spirit of ubuntu: Enforcing the rights of orphans and vulnerable children affected by HIV/AIDS in South Africa. *Hastings International and Comparative Law Review, 31*(1), 33–113.

Böhm, D., & Hiley, B. J. (1993). *The undivided universe: An ontological interpretation of quantum theory.* London and New York: Routledge.

CAMH. (2017). *Centre for addiction and mental health.* Retrieved from http://www.camh.ca/en/hospital/Pages/home.aspx. Accessed 15th May 2017.

Chan, C. W., Wong, F. K. Y., Yeung, S. M., & Sum, F. (2016). Holistic health status questionnaire: Developing a measure from a Hong Kong Chinese population. *Health and Quality of Life Outcomes, 14*(1), 28.

Christakis, N. A. (2012). Holism. In J. Brockman (Ed.), *This will make you smarter* (pp. 81–83). New York: Harper.

Comprehensive School Health. (2017). *Pan Canadian joint consortium for school health.* http://www.jcsh-cces.ca/index.php/about/comprehensive-school-health. Accessed 13th May 2017.

Dahlgren, G., & Whitehead, M. (1991). *Policies and strategies to promote social equity in health.* Stockholm, Sweden: Institute for Future Studies. Retrieved from http://eurohealthnet.eu/sites/eurohealthnet.eu/les/publications/DETERMINE-Final-Publication-Story.pdf. Accessed 24th April 2017.

Descartes, R. (1998). *The world and other writings* (S. Gaukroger, Trans.). Cambridge: Cambridge University Press. (Original work published 1664).

de Silva, D. (2014). *Helping measure person-centred care: A review of evidence about commonly used approaches and tools used to help measure person-centred care.* London: The Health Foundation.

Downing, C., & Hastings-Tolsma, M. (2016). An integrative review of Albertina Sisulu and ubuntu: Relevance to caring and nursing. *Health sa Gesondheid, 21, 214–227.*

Edwards, S., Makunga, N., Ngcobo, S., & Dhlomo, M. (2004). Ubuntu: A cultural method of mental health promotion. *International Journal of Mental Health Promotion, 6*(4), 17–22. doi:10.1080/14623730.2004.9721940.

Einstein, A. (1936). *Letter from Einstein to Smuts, June 24: Volume 54.* Cambridge: Cambridge University Library.

English Oxford Living Dictionary. (2016). *Holism.* Retrieved from https://en.oxforddictionaries.com/definition/holism.

Freeman, J. (2005). Towards a definition of holism. *The British Journal of General Practice, 55* (511), 154–155.

Fullerton, J. (2015). *Regenerative capitalism: How universal principles and patterns will shape our new economy.* Capital Institute. Retrieved from http://capitalinstitute.org/wp-content/uploads/2015/04/2015-Regenerative-Capitalism-4-20-15-final.pdf.

Graham, H., & Leeseberg-Stamler, L. (2010). Contemporary perceptions from an Indigenous (plains cree) perspective. *Journal of Aboriginal Health, 6, 6–17.*

Griffiths, P. (1988, January 3). An Indigenous philosophy of living. *Daily Herald-Rural Roots.* Retrieved from http://www.libraries.gov.sk.ca/booksinfo/DailyHerald/DH1988/dh880123.html.

Hancock, T., & Perkins, F. (1985). The mandala of health: A conceptual model and teaching tool. *Health Education, 24*(1), 8–10.

Harkin, M. E. (2010). Uncommon ground: Holism and the future of anthropology. *Reviews in Anthropology, 39*(1), 25–45.

Harrington, A. (1996). *Reenchanted science: Holism in German culture from Wilhelm II to Hitler.* Princeton, NJ: Princeton University Press.

Hunter, L. M., Logan, J., Goùlet, J., & Barton, S. (2006). Aboriginal healing: Regaining balance and culture. *Journal of Transcultural Nursing, 17*(1), 13–22.

Indigenous Physicians Association of Canada & The Association of Faculties of Medicine of Canada (IPAC & AFMC). (2009). *First nations, Inuit, Metis health: Core competencies: A curriculum framework for undergraduate medical education.* Retrieved from https://afmc.ca/sites/default/files/documents/en/Medical-Education/Aboriginal-Health-Needs/CoreCompetenciesEng.pdf.

Isberg, R. R., & Falkow, S. (1985). A single genetic locus encoded by *Yersinia pseudotuberculosis* permits invasion of cultured animal cells by *Escherichia coli* K-12. *Nature, 317*(6034), 262–264.

Járos, G. (2002). Holism revisited: Its principles 75 years on. *World Futures, 58*(1), 13–32.

Katinić, M. (2013). Holism in deep ecology and Gaia-theory: A contribution to eco-geological science, a philosophy of life or a new age stream? *The Holistic Approach to Environment, 3*(1), 3–14.

Kendell, R. (2001). The distinction between mental and physical illness. *The British Journal of Psychiatry, 178,* 490–493.

Khenti, A., Fréel, S., Trainor, R., Mohamoud, S., Diaz, P., Suh, E., … Sapag, J. C. (2015). Developing a holistic policy and intervention framework for global mental health. *Health Policy and Planning, 31*(1), 37–45.

Kitano, H. (2002). Systems biology: A brief overview. *Science, 295*(5560), 1662–1664.

Kitching, R. L. (1983). *Systems ecology: An introduction to ecological modelling.* St. Lucia, Australia: University of Queensland Press.

Lundh, L. (2015). Combining holism and interactionism: Towards a conceptual clarification. *Journal for Person-Oriented Research, 1*(3), 185–194.

Marston, J. M. (2015). The spirit of "ubuntu" in children's palliative care. *Journal of Pain and Symptom Management, 50*(3), 424–427.

Michaelson, V., Pickett, W., King, N., & Davison, C. (2016). Testing the theory of holism: A study of family systems and adolescent health. *Preventive Medicine Reports, 4,* 313–319.

Mulaudzi, M., Libster, M., & Phiri, S. (2009). Suggestions for creating a welcoming nursing community: Ubuntu, cultural diplomacy, and mentoring. *International Journal for Human Caring, 13*(2), 45–51.

National Collaborating Centre for Aboriginal Health (NCCAH). (2013). *Messages from the heart: Caring for our children: A national showcase on Aboriginal child rearing.* Prince George, BC: University of British Columbia. Retrieved from http://www.nccah-ccnsa.ca/Publications/Lists/Publications/Attachments/33/MFTH_EN_web.pdf. Accessed 24th April 2017.

Odum, H. T. (1994). *Ecological and general systems.* Boulder, CO: University Press of Colorado.

Online Etymology Dictionary. (2017). *Holism.* Retrieved from http://etymonline.com/index.php?allowed_in_frame=0&search=holism. Accessed 24th April 2017.

Ontario Ministry of Education. (2015). *The Ontario curriculum grades 1–8: Health and physical education.* Retrieved from http://www.edu.gov.on.ca/eng/curriculum/elementary/health1to8.pdf.

Pan Canadian Joint Consortium for School Health. (2017). http://www.jcsh-cces.ca/. Accessed 13th May 2017.

Phillips, D. C. (1976). *Holistic thought in social science.* Stanford, CA: Stanford University Press.

Plato. (380 BCE). *Charmides.* Retrieved from http://classics.mit.edu/Plato/charmides.html. Accessed 24th April 2017.

Scott, A. J., & Wilson, R. F. (2011). Peer reviewed: Upstream ecological risks for overweight and obesity among African American youth in a rural town in the deep south, 2007. *Preventing Chronic Disease, 8*(1): A17.

Smuts, J. C. (1926). *Holism and evolution.* Рипол Классик.

Stempsey, W. E. (2001). Plato and holistic medicine. *Medicine, Health Care and Philosophy, 4*(2), 201–209.

Strong, J. (2005). Shalom.7965. Strong's Exhaustive Concordance. Retrieved from http://biblehub.com/hebrew/7965.htm. Accessed 24 April 2017.

Svenson, K., & Lafontaine, C. (1999). The search for wellness. In G. McDonald (Ed.), *First Nations and Inuit regional health survey national report* (181–216). Retrieved from http://uregina.ca/library/holdings/FN_Inuit_Health_Survey.pdf. Accessed 24 April 2017.

Swanson, R. C., Cattaneo, A., Bradley, E., Chunharas, S., Atun, R., Abbas, K. M., ... & Best, A. (2012). Rethinking health systems strengthening: Key systems thinking tools and strategies for transformational change. *Health Policy and Planning, 27*(suppl 4), iv54–iv61.

Sweat, M. D., & Denison, J. A. (1995). Reducing HIV incidence in developing countries with structural and environmental interventions. *Aids, 9,* S251–S257.

Tagalik, S. (2010). *Inuit qaujimajatuqangit: The role of Indigenous knowledge in supporting wellness in Inuit communities in Nunavut.* Prince George, BC: National Collaborating Center for Aboriginal Health. Retrieved from http://www.nccah-ccnsa.ca/docs/child%20and%20youth/Indigenous%20Knowledge%20in%20Inuit%20Communities%20(English%20-%20web).pdf. Accessed 24 April 2017.

WHO. (1986a). *Healthy settings.* Geneva: World Health Organization. Retrieved from http://www.who.int/healthy_settings/en/. Accessed 24 April 2017.

WHO. (1986b). *Ottawa charter for health promotion.* Proceedings from the First International Conference on Health Promotion. Ottawa, ON: World Health Organization. Retrieved from http://www.euro.who.int/en/publications/policy-documents/ottawa-charter-for-health-promotion,-1986. Accessed 24 April 2017.

WHO. (1992). *The ICD-10 classification of mental and behavioural disorders: Clinical descriptions and diagnostic guidelines.* Geneva: World Health Organization. Retrieved from http://apps.who.int/classifications/icd10/browse/2010/en. Accessed 24 April 2017.

WHO. (2007). *People-centred health care: A policy framework.* Geneva: World Health Organization. Retrieved from http://www.wpro.who.int/health_services/people_at_the_centre_of_care/documents/ENG-PCIPolicyFramework.pdf. Accessed 24 April 2017.

WHO. (2009). *Milestones in health promotion: Statements from global conferences.* Retrieved from http://www.who.int/healthpromotion/milestones/en/. Accessed April 24, 2017.

Wollumbin, J. (2012). Holistic primary health care: Origins and history. *Journal of the Australian traditional medicine society, 18,* 77–80.

Zelko, F. (2012). A mind divided against itself: Thinking holistically with a split brain. *Environment, Culture, and the Brain: New Explorations In Neurohistory, 6,* 17–22.

Chapter 2
Child Perceptions of Health

Health is not simply a definition. It can't just be something in a dictionary, it's more complicated than that.
—Focus group participant

This Convention encourages adults to listen to the opinions of children….
—Convention on the Rights of the Child, Article 12

Abstract In this chapter, we intentionally listen to the opinions and ideas of children in order to understand the potential value or relevance, if any, of holism to child health. We present findings from a 2014 qualitative study with children from across Ontario, Canada. This novel study aimed to describe young people's perceptions of health. Several key findings emerged: (1) Children found standard definitions about health useful but limited in value; (2) Children wanted a model of health that was flexible enough to be "different for everyone"; (3) All the "different for everyone" aspects of health are interconnected; (4) Metaphors such as a cake, a house, a web and a maze were proposed by the children as useful ways of talking about health, and may offer a flexible, practical, holistic and fresh framework for engaging with children about health; and (5) Metaphors are a useful technique for engaging children with the abstract concept of holism.

Keywords Holism · Qualitative research · Metaphors · Perceptions of health · Generational theory

Ask an adult what health is, and she may tell you one thing. Ask a child, and you may hear something entirely different.

In Chap. 1 of this book, we discussed the idea of holism as having potential value for many aspects of child health. We saw this value reflected in school curricula as well as frameworks such as Comprehensive School Health (CSC, 2017), which is championed by the Pan Canadian Joint Consortium of School Health (2017). We also saw this idea reflected in key health promotion frameworks, notably in the Ottawa Charter (WHO, 1986). These approaches encourage us to make connections between the domains of health within an individual, but also to

© The Author(s) 2018
V. Michaelson et al., *Holistic Health in Children: Conceptualization, Assessment and Potential*, SpringerBriefs in Well-Being and Quality of Life Research, DOI 10.1007/978-3-319-64831-6_2

recognize the interdependence of issues such as social justice, human rights, sustainability and technology with human health. Holistic ideas such as these are informing practice in various contexts around the world.

As much as we recognize the strength of these approaches, we also identified a challenge: how can we apply the theory of holism to health in a way that is meaningful to children? We believe that in order to truly be useful to contemporary children, any application of this theory to child health may benefit from consideration of real children in the context of their everyday lives. It is also important to pay attention to people's subjective experiences related to health because people themselves (including children) often have the greatest insight into their own health status and experiences (Lawton, 2003).

All of the voices so far have been those of adults, and the reality is that today's children may conceptualize important components of health in ways that do not fit with past paradigms envisioned by adults. As adult researchers whose work relates to child populations, one of our challenges is "to abandon the commonly held assumption that adults' knowledge is superior to that of children" (Alderson & Goodey, 1996). This relates to what Fletcher describes as "adultism", an agenda that involves prioritizing the beliefs, actions, attitudes and ideas of adults over young people and the favouring of adults by dismissing young people and their energy and ideas (Fletcher, 2015). However, if we do this, and only listen to adult voices, our research is impoverished and we will very likely miss out on important insights and concerns. The most useful way forward is to balance our adult knowledge with reports of children's own perspectives and experiences.

In the next two chapters, we intentionally listen to the opinions and ideas of children in order to understand the potential value or relevance, if any, of holism to child health. We do this by presenting findings from a 2014 qualitative study with children from across Ontario, Canada that aimed to describe young people's perceptions of health. In Chap. 3, we present a second (2016/17) and complementary qualitative study that builds on what was learned from the first.

Child Perceptions of Health: A Qualitative Study

Qualitative research methods are used to gather information or data that is not in numerical form, in order to provide rich accounts of human perceptions and experiences. They are a powerful way to gain understanding about complex issues and human experiences.

Using a focus group method, we compiled a range of stories and insights about children's experiences of health. Participants in our qualitative study were 40 girls and boys between the ages of 11 and 15, organized in seven focus groups from a mix of rural and urban locations throughout Ontario, Canada. Rather than engage these children in a philosophical discussion about holism, our goal was to engage them in thinking about what would make up the health of a whole person. We were curious if they would tell us that there were certain components that should be included, or if some aspects of health were more important than others. We wondered if thinking about health in this way would even resonate with this population group, or if a more reductionist or compartmentalized approach would be easier to understand. Various techniques were used to elicit ideas. The full methods for this study are reported in Appendix A and here we primarily report and discuss our results.

Definitions of Health

We began by showing the children four standard definitions of health, and asked them to choose the definition of health that resonated with them most. Examples included the WHO standard definition of health (WHO, 1948), as well as the "medicine wheel" that remains foundational to Indigenous thinking (Svenson & Lafontaine, 1999). This exercise turned out to be a challenge for all the participants, who overall shared the view that the definitions were not necessarily bad but that they did not fully capture their ideas about health. One participant summed up what seemed to reflect the overarching consensus in all groups: "Health is not simply a definition. It can't just be something in a dictionary, it's more complicated than that".

Modelling Health Step 1: "What Does Health Look like in a Whole Person?"

After this initial discussion about definitions, we asked participants to imagine what health would look like "in a whole person". Using picture cards to fuel discussion, participants engaged in lively discussions, and readily came up with many (depending on the group, 30–40) aspects of health that they thought were important to a whole person. Most groups included aspects like physical activity, social and mental health, nutrition and sleep. Other ideas emerged that we did not necessarily expect, including "being skilled", "having ability", "music" and "having potential". We were told that a healthy person "isn't hunched over" and that "they feel comfortable with themselves".

The focus group participants' ideas were thoughtful, sophisticated and nuanced. One 13 year old told us: "I know someone who has a disease where their hair falls out; but they exercise a lot and they are a happy person. I think that I would consider them a healthy person but they are a sick healthy person". While participants readily described health as having a diversity of constituent parts, there was no consensus as to what the various aspects of health in a whole person would be. Repeatedly, and without exception, children in every group told us that "everyone is different". Thus, any model that reflected positive, holistic health for one person would need to be adapted for the next person because "health is different for everyone".

Modelling Health Step 2: Organizing the Aspects of Health into Categories

The next step in our study was to ask participants to organize the various aspects of health into different categories that would reflect the health of a whole person, and to give each category a descriptive name. Each group approached this task in a slightly different manner. Most groups had a category simply called "physical health". Some of their categories related to supportive systems, such as family, peers and schools. One group named a group of pictures they thought connected to relaxation as a "zen mode". Another group wanted to distinguish between positive mental health and barriers to mental health. They called one category "positive mental" and another "twisted ideals mental," which they told us reflected mental health struggles related to social pressures around body image. Each group wound up with a unique set of categories of health (usually 4–7) that they thought were important to the overall health of a person (though precisely what aspects would go into each category was never fully established).

Modelling Health Step 3: Organizing the Categories into the Health of a Whole Person

After the categories were established, we transcribed the names of each category onto 8-inch translucent circles. We then invited participants to organize the circles into a model that would "show us what health looks like all together in a whole person their age". It was here that another real challenge began. While there was a great deal of animated discussion, the only thing that was agreed upon was that this modelling could not be done. This was because, as the children had repeatedly said, everyone is different. And so, how the categories would go together in a person would be "different for everyone" too. As one person put it:

> Different people need different amounts of each one. It depends on who you are and what you need to be healthy. Some people want more time with other people and that makes them feel healthier and then some people want more time by themselves and that makes them feel healthier. It depends on the person.

However the parts went together, the children did agree on a few key things: health has many components, and all the component parts are interrelated and vital to the whole. As one participant told us, "Every category of health ties in with the others". Another said "No matter how you categorize them they will be interconnected and a lot of people will experience all of them and they will all tie into one thing". Not only are all the components interconnected, but "… if we take one thing out, everything else suffers".

Figures 2.1 and 2.2 are illustrative examples of the models that were made in two different groups.

Fig. 2.1 Organizing categories of health, model 1

Fig. 2.2 Organizing
categories of health, model 2

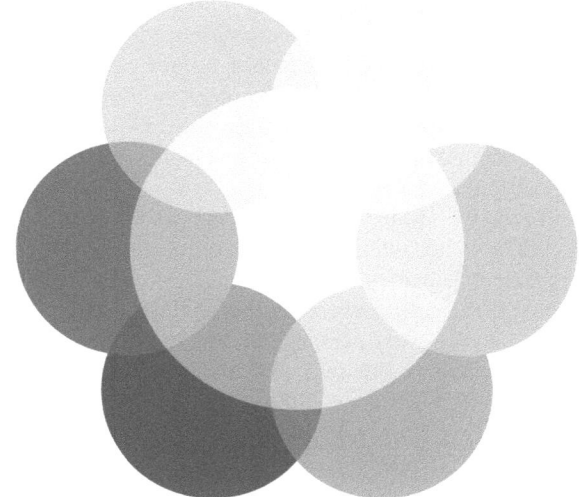

This idea about the interdependence between the parts was very much in keeping with the framework for holistic health that we presented in Chap. 1. And yet, upon reflection, we realized that we needed to interpret this with caution. We had intentionally asked our participants to consider what health looks like in a whole person, and so it makes sense that they would respond with a holistic, interconnected model. Had we asked for a reductionist model, they might just as easily have responded with such. Because of this, we cannot conclude from this study that young people naturally view health in holistic ways. What our study does suggest, however, is that holistic and integrated ways of thinking about health resonate well with this age group.

Health Is Different for Everyone?

One of our goals was to discover a useful and practical way of using holistic thinking to talk about health with young people that would resonate with their own experiences. What these qualitative findings showed us was that any model or framework for holistic health that we developed would have to recognize the unique context, needs and health status of each child.

On reflection, this is perhaps not a surprise, and is in keeping with contemporary generational theory. The children who participated in our study were all born at the end of the 1990s or early 2000s. They are at the early end of what some have described as the iGeneration (Rosen, 2010; Wood et al., 2013). The "i" represents not only the type of technologies used by this group (iTunes, iPhones, iPads, etc.), but also reflects the highly individualized activities and profiles that are facilitated by these technologies. Wood et al., (2013) reflect on characteristics of this generation in the realm of healthcare, writing: "If music, television, advertising, and internet search engines can be customized and available in a click or a tap, then the same expectation will be placed upon healthcare" (p. 1). The refrain "health is different for everyone" also reflects a trend in this population group toward inclusivity (Jonas-Dwyer & Pospisil, 2004). If positive health is truly viewed as different for everyone, then each person's health state can be viewed as normative and no one is left out.

There was little agreement amongst our participants about what components would go into a holistic model of health, or how those components would be organized. But they did agree on this: any model of health that will work for children their age needs to be inclusive and customized, and recognize the uniqueness of every person. Our challenge, then, was to find a way of talking about and modeling health that was malleable, and that could adapt to each person's health state, behaviours, ideas and context. We needed something concrete yet flexible. This was a tall order.

And yet, an unexpected and innovative idea emerged early on, straight from our participants. How about using metaphors to talk about health?

Using Metaphors as a Framework for Talking About Health

A metaphor is a comparison; it is a way of showing how two distinct things that are not alike in most ways are similar in another important way. The metaphor may provide clarity, or offer insight into similar ideas between them. Here is an example. Saying an idea is "food for thought" doesn't mean that an idea will quite literally be eaten. It is a metaphor about an idea being substantial enough to provide cognitive or intellectual nourishment. In this and similar ways, metaphors are powerful tools for fostering understanding between two conceptual domains. Typically, one of the domains is more abstract (like "ideas" or, in our case, "health") while the other is more concrete (like "food") (Lakoff & Johnson, 1980).

The idea of using metaphors to talk about holistic health was unanticipated by our research team. Indeed, the idea of using metaphors had emerged two or three times in our focus groups before we began to give it due attention. While the participants did not discount the definitions or models, they were unanimous in their enthusiasm for using the metaphors as the most helpful vehicle for talking about health because as one participant told us, "they are easier to compare and see how they relate and how they connect". When we discussed the definitions of health, we constantly had to prompt the children to share their ideas. However, when the metaphors were introduced, the energy in the groups changed. Participants shared creatively, and readily made connections to their own lives.

In the next section, we report some of the initial ideas that the young people shared about how metaphors could be used to think about the health of a whole person.

Health Is a Cake

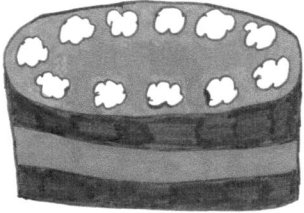

In our first focus group, participants were having an engaging discussion about the different components that make up the health of a whole person. Here is the conversation that transpired.

First participant   *"You need all of those [different parts] to be healthy. It keeps you all together or something like that. You need all of them… if you are baking something you need everything to be the best it can".*

Second participant   *"Expanding on the metaphor…sometimes you won't have all those so you might have to make adjustments to the recipe but that is okay and it might turn out. It might be a surprise… Every person has a different recipe of their life. Some people have…".*

Third participant   *"Different priorities….".*

We were intrigued with this metaphor and presented it to subsequent groups as a potential way of talking about health. The children responded to this idea with enthusiasm, and shared many ideas about ways of thinking about a cake that they found helpful in understanding health. In one group, a child told us that there are "so many components that need to be together to make one really good thing". Others had all kinds of ideas about what the ingredients of a good health cake would be: physical, mental, and social well-being; respect, emotional health, water, sleep, food, friends, exercise and family. One boy shared that happiness would go into his cake, as a way of supporting his emotional and mental health. And another shared that people with physical challenges or diseases would need "extra ingredients in their cake" to help them because "when you have cancer it takes down your energy and you have other things to think about".

It didn't take long before the "different for everyone" priority was applied to the metaphors. In one group, participants were discussing social health, and we asked if that would be an ingredient in a health cake. One person replied:

> I think if you are happy without being social then that is like okay …being social would not make everyone happy. So if it makes you happy then I think it needs to be a part of it but if you are fine with being on your own and not being social then I don't think it needs to be a part of it.

Another person told us that everyone has "a different recipe for their life". Our challenge had been to find a way of talking about health with young people that was concrete (and focussed on health), but also allowed for flexibility. The metaphor of health as a cake had accomplished this.

There was depth and nuance to the conversation, and participants in this group were adamant that a health cake does not necessarily have only good things in it. We asked them to say more about this:

First participant   *You don't live a life without unhappy things. I have never met somebody that everything good happens to them like I won the lottery and oh I won it again. You always have disappointments in your life….*

Second participant   *I have never met someone who has never been sad basically or unhappy.*

We asked how this related to a health cake and were told it would be reflected in the colours and the different layers:

Second participant   *If you are unhappy [the bottom layer] would be black… some people are always unhappy because of depression and stuff like that and then half or more of the cake would be black.*

This theme of health as a cake, and the opportunity to discuss the ingredients in their own health cake, captivated this group, and gave them a framework for exploring creative new perspectives and ideas about health.

Health Is a House

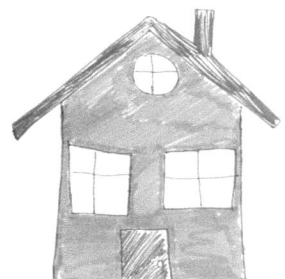

The house metaphor was suggested in our second group, and inspired just as lively a conversation as the cake. Children described all sorts of different materials that would make up a healthy house, including social well-being, and mental and physical health. Friends and family would be the "walls to hold the house up" and healthy eating and exercise would be "maybe the roof or the halls and the doors". One child told us that "you need to have emotions in your health so maybe the lights would be sadness" and another said that for her, "lights would be happiness. I am not sure if it is a simile or metaphor but one moment of kindness can change a person's day".

Participants spent a good amount of time discussing the foundation of the house, one participant claiming that it "would be the most important part". For one child, the foundation would be "healthy/active living and mental and emotional health". Another boy told us that the foundation of his house would include "happiness and all the good parts" while a girl said "I like the idea that mental health is the ground and floor and the people are the walls".

The idea of the interconnected nature of health emerged strongly with this house metaphor. One child reflected that "*If you are missing some components, which is like a brick, then your house won't be as steady*". Another told us this:

> Your walls could be made of glass so beautiful on the outside but can break really easily. So if it breaks the whole thing could shatter and then drop. So if one strand is compromised then it has the ability to bring down the whole house. If the foundation is compromised then the house has nothing to stand on. And I think the house really illuminates that idea of staying strong and what everything is made out of.

Again, just as when young people in focus groups talked about the baking and the cake, it was the young people's ideas that drove the conversation and they genuinely seemed to enjoy thinking about health in this way.

Health Is a Maze

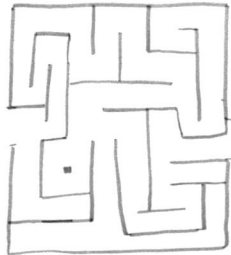

New metaphors continued to emerge, and in the third focus group, the idea of health as a maze was introduced.

First participant | *To me [health] looks like a maze and you have to go through the maze to get to the end. You start at the very beginning of your health spot and get to your goal by the end of the maze.*
Second participant | *And there are obstacles in the middle and you have to overcome challenges and obstacles...*
Third participant | *So to get to the end to get to where you want to be...." (We asked "What is at the end of your maze?")...Like what your goal is and what you want to be and what you want to achieve.*

For these children, it was clearly important to discuss obstacles. One girl told us that "if you are trying to get fit and eat healthy then there are certain days where you just completely forget about doing it and that would be an obstacle day of the maze". We were curious about what was meant by "obstacle day" and when we probed, several different participants shared ideas. The first child told us that obstacles could be "depression" or "being upset". One boy was particularly interested in talking about obstacles related to health that you would find in your maze. He said "when the obstacles come you can choose to get back up or to stay down in self-pity when you get knocked down".

The health maze metaphor discussion revealed diverse ideas that we had not yet heard. For example, one person had an idea about challenging yourself to think about how you handle your own health: "The walls could be different parts or questions in the maze. Like you have to pass a question to move on". The question might be: "How do you deal with mental health?" or "Are you physically active?".

For another participant, there was a progressive element to the maze:

> *Health is a maze. It is like when you first start off it is easy and you know what to do and then it gets harder. So when I first started to eat healthy or act healthy it is easy to think, I am going to do this and this. But then it gets harder like a maze. When you are going through a maze it gets harder.*

As researchers, we were very curious about this maze metaphor, and wondered what they thought that they needed to navigate their health maze well, or to find their way out. One youth responded "A strong adult that you would trust".

Health Is a Web

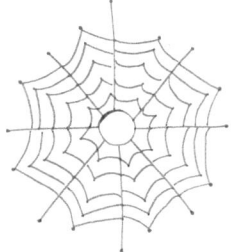

The final metaphor to emerge from this series of focus groups was a web. One child used this image to describe the way all of health is "intertwined". Another told us that all parts of health "tie in altogether. You do sports with your friends too so you have your physical side and your mental side". The observation that different aspects of health are interconnected continued in a subsequent group: "All the parts have to fit together in a certain way so…you have to make sure that your activity corresponds to what you eat so …if you are doing a lot of activity you have to eat a lot and it all connects together".

While we have fewer illustrative examples of how young people used the web, we suspect that this is not because it was less meaningful than the other three metaphors but rather, that it emerged in one of the later groups. One girl who chose the web as her favourite of the four metaphors saw it as a way of connecting every part of health together "by one main thing, kind of". But what the one main thing would be, of course, she told us, "might be different for everyone".

Summary Insights About Metaphors

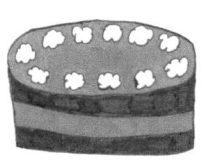 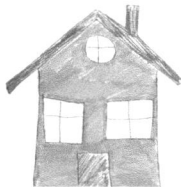 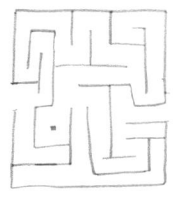 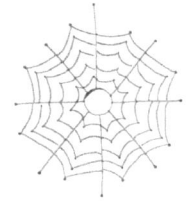

By the final focus group, four metaphors for health had emerged directly from our discussions: the cake, the house, the maze and the web. New and creative ideas developed with each metaphor and alternative and creative perspectives about health emerged. Once we recognized how deeply the metaphor theme was res-onating with focus participants, we began asking the young people to vote on which metaphor they preferred. The votes were nearly always evenly split between the four metaphors (with many of the participants telling us "I like all of them"). Several of the participants told us that all the metaphors were connected, and one even went so far as to say "all your metaphors mean the same thing".

We were encouraged by how readily the young people engaged with the metaphors, and how much they seemed to enjoy the discussions. One child told us this:

> I wanted to say that this exercise is really cool.... It is cool to see different people's perspectives... to see different people with different beliefs and styles than me. It is cool to see everyone organizing and explaining why and I can see why everybody does everything but it is like they... they all have something that changes and makes them different than everybody else. It is nice to see that.

For the participants in our study, the real value seemed to be that each metaphor provided a framework for discussion that was concrete yet flexible, and that afforded everyone the freedom to develop the metaphor with respect to their own unique experiences. Recall Lakoff and Johnson's (1980) idea that one part of a metaphor is generally concrete (like a house or a cake) while the other is more abstract (like holistic health). It is the concrete side of the metaphor that provided a shared and familiar framework. The house, for example, was familiar to all participants; there was a general consensus that a house should have a foundation, a door, a roof, windows, and lights. When put together with the more abstract idea of health, alternative and creative perspectives were formed. The house was concrete, yet it was also abstract and flexible enough that it could still look different for every person.

Metaphors became a vivid way of facilitating the young people to think deeply about health and to dialogue with others about their ideas. Whereas definitions had offered bounded structure, metaphors had offered a conceptual framework that became a starting point for a dynamic discussion. Through metaphor, the laboratory of health science was connected to their real, human lives.

We return to Lakoff and Johnson, whose groundbreaking work in this area has demonstrated that we are wired to understand concepts metaphorically, and that concepts that are abstract or more complex (for example, health) become better understood in relation to more familiar concepts. In other words, metaphors help us take what we know about something that is known (such as a house or cake) and from that prior knowledge, move to better understanding about what is unknown (Lakoff & Johnson, 1980). Metaphors can function as a kind of "cognitive shortcut" that can help children to understand complex ideas. Mabeck and Oleson (1996) take this argument even further and suggest that metaphors go beyond describing similarities (health and a cake both have ingredients) to creating new ideas (Mabeck & Oleson, 1996). When "this" is like "that", each conceptual category informs the other, and new, alternative and creative perspectives are formed. In retrospect, it is logical that metaphors from their everyday lives helped the children in our study to form new ideas about their health.

The use of metaphors in health settings is not a new idea. A powerful discussion of the ways that metaphors are used in the discourse on cancer is given by Resifield and Wilson (2004). In another context, a football metaphor was used to engage men in mental health services (Spandler, Roy, & Mckeown, 2014). In the UK, the metaphor of the family was used to help practitioners understand the new responsibilities and challenges that came about because of changes to primary health care (Warne & Stark, 2003). The house metaphor was used to help in delivering better services for people with long term conditions (Coulter, Roberts, & Dixon, 2013) and the "Man Manual" (Banks, 2002), designed to mimic a car maintenance manual, uses the metaphor of the biological body as a machine to promote men's health. Our study led us to realize that metaphors may have value too for engaging children in considering their own health.

We began this chapter by suggesting that child paradigms of health might be quite different from those constructed by adults. This new generation may not operate within older structures and logic, and in order to truly engage with today's young people, we suggest that new frameworks for talking about health may be required. When we asked the young people to react to standard definitions of health, they gave us simple responses without much depth. However, when we invited them to interact with this idea of health as a metaphor, they were creative and engaged. Talking about health using metaphors appears to be a fresh and useful framework that resonates well with today's young people. Metaphors were useful and dynamic tools for sparking conversations around health and helped the young people to organize their ideas in new and creative ways.

Another advantage of using metaphors is that they are flexible. In one participant's house, for example, the lights represented happiness but for another, they symbolized being sad. What seemed important was not that each component of a house (or any of the other metaphors) had a direct parallel with health, but that the metaphor gave young people a way of talking about health that left room for the diversity and uniqueness of each person. This framework was flexible enough to allow for the idea that "health is different for everyone" and to allow for young people's own subjective ideas to emerge. A "one-size-fits-all" approach is not going to be helpful for health promotion efforts that target this population.

Bridging Back to Holism

By using metaphors, we discovered a flexible framework to engage in important conversations about health with young people. Metaphors have been a valuable tool to respect the ideas of children. These ideas are a necessary and vital springboard to the main purpose of this book, which is to apply basic principles of the theory of holism to many aspects of child health.

We want to do this in a way that resonates with and is meaningful to children, and that provides new insights that can inform children's health in a variety of ways. We also want to do this in a way that supports the kind of holistic initiatives that we discussed in Chap. 1. For example, our initial exercise that had children determine different categories, or domains, of health was in keeping with the

Ontario Curriculum's goal of encouraging students to make connections between different aspects of their health, including physical, mental, spiritual, social and emotional domains. While our traditional, definition-based modeling exercise was frustrating for the children, when they began to explore the connections between the different categories using metaphors, the conversation was much richer, and the children were visibly excited by their own ideas. Further, their ideas reflected the two defining properties of holism that we presented in the last chapter: the whole is bigger than the sum of the parts (new ideas emerge that are not present when looking at the individual parts); and, the parts are interdependent, and gain new meaning when they are considered in relation to the whole.[1] Metaphors provide an intriguing framework for achieving this goal of talking about health holistically with children. The objective of the next chapter is to test this idea further.

Key Insights from This Chapter

- The Convention on the Rights of the Child (1989) states that if children are being studied, they have a right to have a voice in matters that concern them
- Children's perceptions about health and associated needs might be different from those of adults
- Listening intentionally to the ideas and perspectives of children provides new opportunities to develop meaningful ways of engaging with children in conversations about health

Key Findings

- We conducted a qualitative study in order to understand children's perceptions of holistic health

  - Children found standard definitions about health useful but limited in value
  - Children wanted a model of health that was flexible enough to be "different for everyone"

---

[1]To argue that these metaphors are holistic needs qualification. Think back to Chap. 1, and the first example we gave of holism: the metaphor of a birthday cake. We wrote about how Jan Smuts (the first to popularize the term holism in the early 20th century), made a clear distinction between mechanical systems and true holism (Smuts, 1926). By Smuts' definition, only the cake would be a model of true holism because when the parts are combined, it changes on a metaphysical level (Smuts, 1926). It is no longer "eggs, flour, butter and sugar"; it is something entirely new. The house, the web and maze would all fall under the category of a mechanical system. Consider the many parts of a house. Even when the house is put together, a door is still a door, and a window is still a window. Even when they are a vital part of the whole house, they still maintain their own unique properties. And yet the eggs in the cake are no longer eggs—they are inextricably now cake. For the purposes of using metaphors to talk about health with young people, we argue that a purist form of holism does not matter. The practical value of the metaphors of cake, house, maze and web is high, and therefore should not be discounted because they do not represent what Smuts would consider true holism.

- For the children in our study, all the "different for everyone" aspects of health need to be interconnected
- Metaphors such as a cake, a house, a web and a maze were proposed by the children as useful ways of talking about health, and may offer a flexible, practical, holistic and fresh framework for engaging with children about health
- Metaphors are a useful technique by which one can engage with children about the abstract concept of holism

References

Alderson, P., & Goodey, C. (1996). Research with disabled children: How useful is child-centred ethics? *Children and Society, 10*(2), 106–116.

Banks, I. (2002). *The man manual*. Sparkford, UK: JH Haynes & Co Ltd.

Comprehensive School Health (CSC). (2017). Pan Canadian Joint Consortium for School Health. http://www.jcsh-cces.ca/index.php/about/comprehensive-school-health. Accessed 13th May 2017.

Coulter, A., Roberts, S., & Dixon, A. (2013). *Delivering better services for people with long-term conditions: Building the house of care* (pp. 1–28). London: The King's Fund.

Fletcher, A. (2015). *Facing adultism*. CreateSpace Independent Publishing Platform.

Jonas-Dwyer, D., & Pospisil, R. (2004). *Proceedings from the 2004 annual international conference of the higher education research and development society of Australasia (HERDSA): The millennial effect: Implications for academic development*. Malaysia: Sarawak.

Lakoff, G., & Johnson, M. (1980). *Metaphors we live by*. Chicago: University of Chicago Press.

Lawton, J. (2003). Lay experiences of health and illness: Past research and future agendas. *Sociology of Health & Illness, 25*, 23–40.

Mabeck, C. E., & Oleson, F. (1996). Metaphors and understanding of disease. *Ugeskrift for Laeger, 158*, 7384–7387.

Pan Canadian Joint Consortium for School Health. (2017). http://www.jcsh-cces.ca/. Accessed 13th May 2017.

Preamble to the Constitution of the World Health Organization as adopted by the International Health Conference, New York, 19–22 June, 1946; signed on 22 July 1946 by the representatives of 61 States (Official Records of the World Health Organization, no. 2, p. 100) and entered into force on 7 April 1948.

Resifield, G. M., & Wilson, G. R. (2004). Use of metaphor in the discourse on cancer. *Journal of Clinical Oncology, 19*, 4024–4027.

Rosen, L. D. (2010). *Rewired: Understanding the iGeneration and the way they learn*. New York, NY: Palgrave Macmillan.

Smuts, J. C. (2013). *Holism and evolution*. Gouldsboro, ME: Gestalt Journal Press. (Original work published 1926).

Spandler, H., Roy, A. N., & Mckeown, M. (2014). Using football metaphor to engage men in mental health services. *Journal of Social Work Practice, 28*(2), 229–245.

Svenson, K., & Lafontaine, C. (1999). The search for wellness. In G. McDonald (Ed.), *First Nations and Inuit regional health survey national report* (pp. 181–216). Retrieved from http://uregina.ca/library/holdings/FN_Inuit_Health_Survey.pdf. Accessed 24th April 2017.

Warne, T., & Stark, S. (2003). The family practitioner family: The use of metaphor in understanding changes in primary health care organizations. *Primary Health Care Research & Development, 4*(4), 292–300.

WHO. (1986). *Ottawa charter for health promotion.* Proceedings from the First International Conference on Health Promotion. Ottawa, ON: World Health Organization. Retrieved from http://www.euro.who.int/en/publications/policy-documents/ottawa-charter-for-health-promotion,-1986. Accessed 24 April 2017.

Wood, K. D., Greene, E. M., Franks, R. B., Poole, T. M., Ficzere, C. H., & Johnston, P. E. (2013). The healthcare future for the iGeneration: Integrating the patient and the healthcare system. *Innovations in Pharmacy, 4*(3), Article 122.

Chapter 3
Metaphors and Child Health

New metaphors are capable of creating new understandings and, therefore, new realities.

George Lakoff, Metaphors We Live By

Abstract In this chapter, we present a second (2016/17) and complementary qualitative study, "Using children's drawing of metaphors to explore holistic health", which builds on what was learned from the "Child perceptions of health" study presented in Chap. 2. Participants were asked to draw and then engage with their own metaphor of health. The purpose was to explore more deeply the practical utility of using metaphors for engaging with children about holistic health, and also to explore how adding evidence-based health knowledge to children's initial discussions may stretch and deepen their understanding of their own health. Along with the cake, the house, the web and the maze, two new metaphors were proposed by participants—a Jenga game and a car engine. Participants found the metaphors to be flexible and useful in integrating health information into their own lives. As participants reflected on their own metaphors, their ideas were in keeping with the properties important to holism: (1) New ideas, particularly around balance, emerged that were not present when studying the individual parts; and (2) The parts appeared to gain new meaning in relation to the whole.

Keywords Holism · Metaphors · Arts-based methods

Holistic thinking undoubtedly has many valuable applications to child health. But holism is not a concrete concept, and not the kind of word that you hear among circles of children. This poses a challenge: how can we use the theoretical concept of holism to talk about health with children in meaningful ways that connect with their real-life experiences, and in fact, in a way that they understand?

The goal of this chapter is to move beyond an abstract conversation and toward a practical and useful way of thinking about child health in a holistic manner. Such an integrative approach would include helping children to recognize the interconnectedness of the many domains of health in their own lives, and equipping them to recognize the impact of their choices in life on their overall health. For example, physical activity can contribute to lower anxiety, which in turn can contribute to better sleep; all of these facets of health are interconnected. Recognizing that these connections exist might encourage children to adopt behaviours that promote positive health in all areas of their lives.

In the last chapter, we suggested that metaphors may be a good way of helping children to understand and connect with their own health holistically. The biggest strength of this idea was that it emerged directly from the conversations with children who participated in our study. And the more they developed the idea of using metaphors as a means of talking about health, the more convinced we were that they were on to something important. The idea also seemed conducive to the properties we were looking for related to holism; the whole is bigger than the sum of the parts and the parts are interconnected.

The flexibility of metaphors appears to be another strength. Whether we are talking about a holistic approach to the health of a whole person, or about a whole community, or extending our conversation to include important determinants of health such as economic or social environments, the focus provided by a concrete metaphor is extremely helpful to facilitating a useful conversation. The metaphor of a cake, for example, has a natural and widely understood set of boundaries. It can be used to describe a whole person or a whole community, and if useful, it can be extended equally to include a whole neighbourhood or to focus specifically on a place such as a whole kitchen. The natural boundaries provided by metaphors mediate the liability that we wrote about in Chap. 1: the potential of holism to become so big that we lose our focus.

Metaphors are also flexible enough to allow for the idea that "health is different for everyone". A "one-size-fits-all" approach was clearly not going to work for the children with whom we spoke, and metaphors allowed room for diversity of thought and expression. We saw this commitment to diversity as a positive feature. For example, it challenges the idea that everyone's body should look the same, or that there is only one way to achieve an optimal state of health. Further, this inclusive approach towards health validates and values different personality styles and social needs. Ideas can emerge from both shy and outgoing participants, and also from young people who have conditions such as asthma, allergies, physical disabilities, etc. that have an impact on shaping their approach to health. All of these people can express views of health that account for their unique strengths and challenges.

However, on reflection, the customized approach to health expressed by many children is not without its disadvantages. For example, when the baseline concept of health is different for everyone, it is difficult to advocate for improved states of health to be fostered via targeted health promotion strategies. And it is not clear that young people appreciate the disconnect between their individualized attitudes and opinions about health and health behaviours, and the basic facts that some behaviours—such as smoking or drug use, poor nutrition or social isolation—have a large evidence base for their negative impacts on health.

We tested this potential concern in another study (Michaelson, Pickett, Vandemeer, Taylor, & Davison, 2016). Using a quantitative analysis of a large population health survey, we looked at children who reported that their health was "good" or "excellent" via a longstanding single item measure (Idler & Benyamini, 1997). Among that group of apparently healthy young people, we also examined their self-reports for a number of clearly established positive and negative health states and behaviours. A full 38% did not meet daily recommended physical activity levels for Canadian adolescents, over half had recently participated in negative bullying behaviours, many reported risk-taking behaviours related to substance abuse, and nearly three-quarters of participants reported indicators of poor emotional health. Further, 17% of those reporting good or excellent health status also indicated that they felt "sad or low every day for two weeks in a row". The latter is particularly concerning, as such feelings provide an initial screen for potential suicidal ideation (Shaffer, Fisher, Lucas, Dulcan, & Schwab-Stone, 2000). The disconnect here is that many young people who perceived themselves to have excellent health simultaneously reported behaviours that would not be in keeping with good health. These findings suggest the need for caution in accepting the views of young people in isolation, or as the only way of assessing their health states and behaviours.

Herein lies our challenge: we wanted to find an approach to engaging young people with the concept of holistic health. But if health in their view is different for everyone, how can we find approaches that allow room for uniqueness, creativity and individual expression but also respect evidence-based thinking? Could metaphors be useful in addressing this challenge? To explore this further, we designed a second qualitative study. In the next section, we describe our methods in brief, and then report and discuss our key findings.

Using Children's Drawing of Metaphors to Explore Holistic Health: A Qualitative Study

Brief Methods

In this study, arts-based drawing techniques were used to elicit conversation and to compile new evidence. Based on other studies that have used drawing techniques (Onyango-Ouma, Aagaard-Hansen, & Jensen, 2004; Piko & Bak, 2006; Pridmore & Bendelow, 1995; Psych & Larsen, 2004), we expected that the use of illustrative drawings would enable children to express their ideas at their own level, and provide a helpful springboard for engaging with ideas about holistic health. This method is child-centred, and demonstrates a respect for children and the importance of listening to their views (DiCarlo, Gibbons, Kaminsky, Wright, & Stiles, 2000; Merriman & Guerin, 2006). Participants were girls and boys between the ages of 11 and 15 from Ontario, Canada (n = 19). Data were collected through two focus groups.

On their own, children's drawings are a challenging medium to interpret in a reliable manner (Thomas & Jolley, 1998). Because of this, the transcription of our audio recording became our primary basis for interpretation of the children's work. Here, children described their own drawings in detail, reflected on the different choices they had made, and often commented on the work of their peers. As much as possible, we have reported their ideas verbatim. Overall, the pictures that the children drew were thoughtful, detailed and bursting with originality and life. We wish that we had room in this small book to print all of them. In this chapter, we provide a few illustrative examples, one for each metaphor. We use the children's own words and descriptions, which elucidate some of the unique and varied ways that the children used the different metaphors to think about their own health.

Introducing Metaphors

We began by introducing examples of metaphors to the children ("those sisters are two peas in a pod" or "your room is a disaster area!"), and found that most participants had a familiarity with such expressions. We talked about how metaphors help us to connect two things or concepts that can't instinctively be viewed as the same, yet have something in common. While they are not true in a literal sense, metaphors sometimes help us think about an issue a bit differently, providing new ideas and insights. We started by explaining that a few years previously, some children their age had told us metaphors could be useful ways of talking about health, and had suggested the metaphors of a house, a cake, a web or a maze for this purpose.

We then provided paper and a variety of sizes and colours of felt markers and asked participants to use one of those metaphors (or another metaphor of their own, if they preferred) to "draw their health". We didn't give directions around what we meant by "their health", and if challenged or asked we simply said "however you understand your health, that's what you draw". We told them that they would have multiple chances to discuss, add to and even change their drawings all together if they so chose. The children drew for about 15 min, and we then asked them to share what they had drawn.

Drawing Health Step 1: Draw Your Health

The children drew mazes, houses, webs and cakes, and also a few new metaphors that surprised us (a car engine and a Jenga game). We asked each child to share what they had done, and also took pictures of what we called step 1 of their drawings.

Four children chose to draw a house, two in each of the two focus groups. Figure 3.1 is an illustrative example of one of the children's drawings.

Fig. 3.1 Health is a house
(step 1)

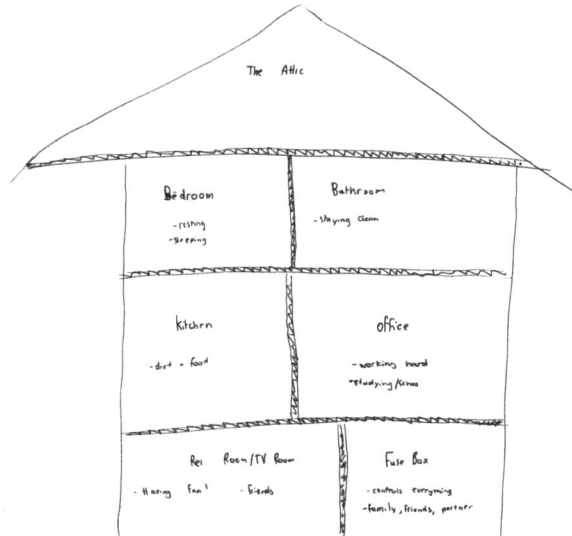

She explained to us what she had been thinking as she drew this metaphor of her health:

> I drew a house and for every room I put what it represents. So the kitchen would be having a healthy diet and the bedroom is resting. There is an office, which is working hard, because you have to work hard for school and stuff. And then I had a TV room because it is important to have fun too. So there is a bit of everything… [I included a fuse box] because I thought there was something in health that controls everything. So kind of like the fuse box. You can turn stuff off and on. So if I decided to turn off all the lights in the bathroom and I was not staying clean anymore then that would be really bad for my health because that would be a part of the house that was not working.

Another child who also had drawn a house told us this:

> I drew a house, the different parts of the house represent different parts of health. Like the windows on my house represent some of the main parts of health for me…. stress with school work, friends, family, homework, etc. The panels on the roof represent different things and if some get pulled out then the roof might fall apart.

Two children drew mazes. Figure 3.2 provides one of their pictures, with a description of what he was thinking about as he drew.

> I think if you take the wrong turn you have to go back just like health. If you eat too much or if you don't get a lot of exercise you have to change what you're doing or where you are going.

The second child who drew a maze also shared her ideas:

> I drew a maze because there are many different routes or paths that you can take. It is not necessarily one path that is right. You can do different things. You can have different dietary plans and you can do other stuff. An example is one path you could take is deciding to run or jog every day.

Fig. 3.2 Health is a maze
(step 1)

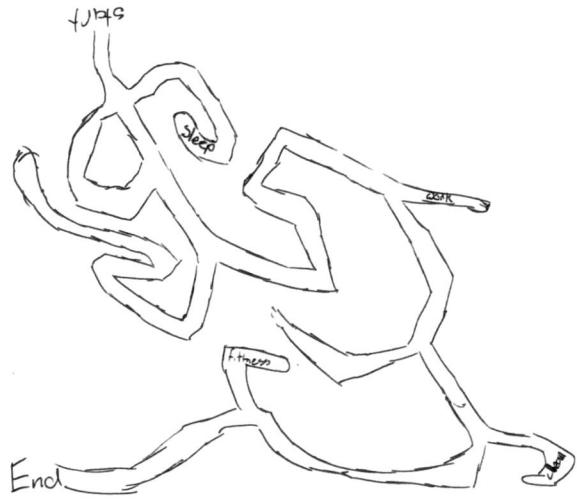

Fig. 3.3 Health is a cake
(step 1)

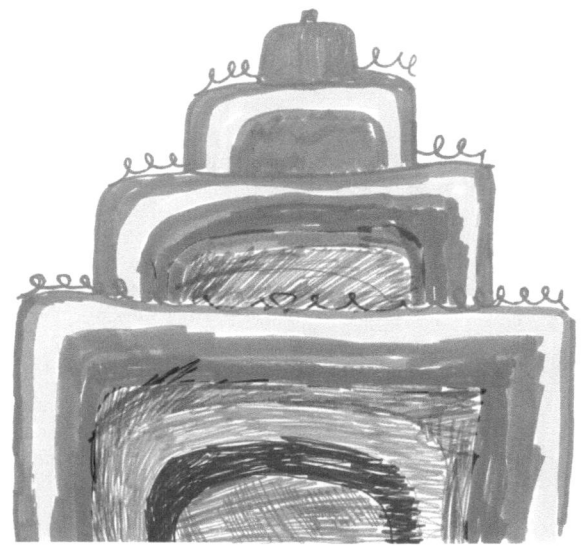

In total, three children drew cakes. The girl who drew the particular cake in Fig. 3.3 described her cake like this:

> I drew a cake with many layers, and the ingredients that go into the cake. The cake represents health, and the ingredients are the things that affect health in a positive or negative.

This idea of "ingredients" came up several times, and we asked the children who had chosen to draw cakes to tell us what kind of ingredients they need in their health cake. One child told us that important ingredients would be "sports and physical activity and staying active. Healthy food and a healthy lifestyle and sleep. And relaxation and not to be stressed out all of the time…". Another told us they would be "nutrition, friends, relaxation, family, sleep, school, and also I do a lot of dance so dance. And then things like art and playing the ukulele because those are creativity and fun".

Two children chose to draw webs, and we share one illustrative picture in Fig. 3.4.

The girl who drew this picture described her drawing like this:

> Mine is a web. I have health and it branched out into mental health, hygiene, oral health, exercise, and nutrition. So then nutrition branches off into healthy diet and getting food from the four food groups. Mental health branches off into good social life and staying happy and stuff and hygiene and washing regularly. So oral health is brushing teeth and flossing. Exercise is exercising on a daily basis and to make sure that you are not always sitting down and doing nothing.

The other child who drew a web told us this:

> I drew sort of a snow flake web thing. The web because the middle point is the starting point and then you have all the options and starting points you can go down. So you make a different choice at every cross web.

Only one child drew a Jenga game. We share his picture in Fig. 3.5 as well as his description of what he drew:

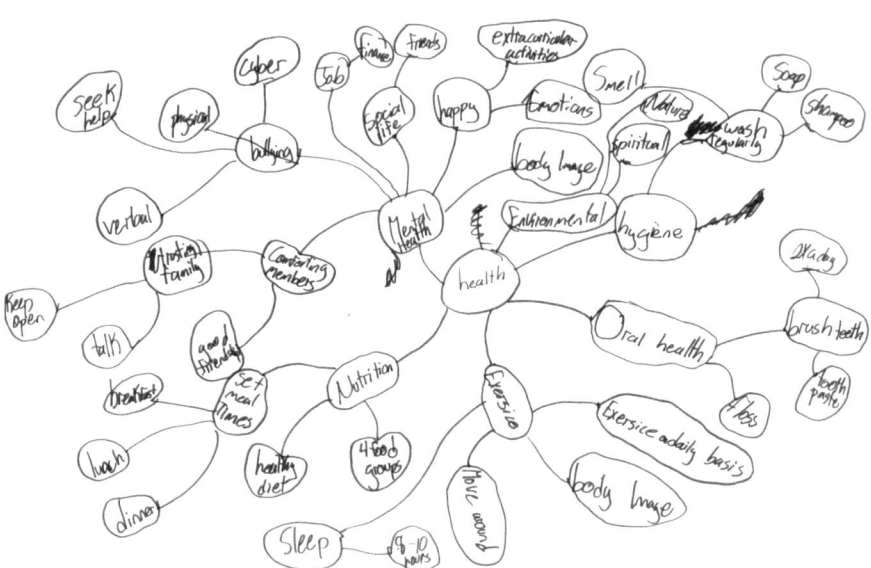

Fig. 3.4 Health is a web (step 1)

Fig. 3.5 Health is a Jenga
game (step 1)

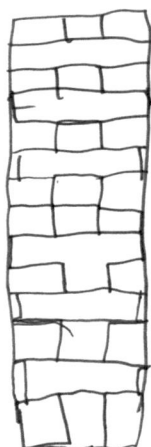

So my poorly drawn drawing that you can't tell what it is…it is actually a Jenga block
tower. I was thinking about how you can take away certain things in your health and
everything and of course the tower will be sturdier with everything in it. But eventually
life…. life is the hand that pulls the blocks out. And it is going to take away some of the
important blocks. And if it takes away too many then your health just crumbles to the
ground. That is kind of what I was thinking. So each block is a different part of your heath
and if too much gets taken away then it will crumble and fall.

We asked him to describe what the various blocks are in his Jenga metaphor of
health.

So school work and homework and everything and that level of stress. So stuff like that. …
school, nutrition….so that can bring out physical health. If you are not eating properly and
are not giving what your body needs then it won't perform properly and your physical
health can drop. School plays in the bigger picture of mental health as well. So mental
health would have a lot of its own blocks which would be stress and family and friends and
relationships. It all balances together to form your mental health and once some of the
things get shaken or taken out then your mental health can crumble as well. That is the same
as your physical health with working out and sleeping and that so your physical health can
also crumble.

Finally, one child drew a car engine (Fig. 3.6).
Here is how he described his drawing.

I did mine as a car's engine. So you can fill it with different parts to make it work. You can
do things to it to make it break down and get destroyed. Everyone keeps saying that there
are a lot of different parts. But I look at it as it is almost like everyone's health has different
engines and different ways they work. So mine might be an American car and someone
else's might be a Chinese car. So it is just how everyone is different. If everyone was the
same then it would be boring. We wouldn't have diversity or anything like that. So each
different part works in a certain way. If that part is taken away then you no longer have it.…
Let's say that you have gasoline then you can put that in the car and it will make it work for
sure. And then a little while later, oh well you need an oil change and you need to change

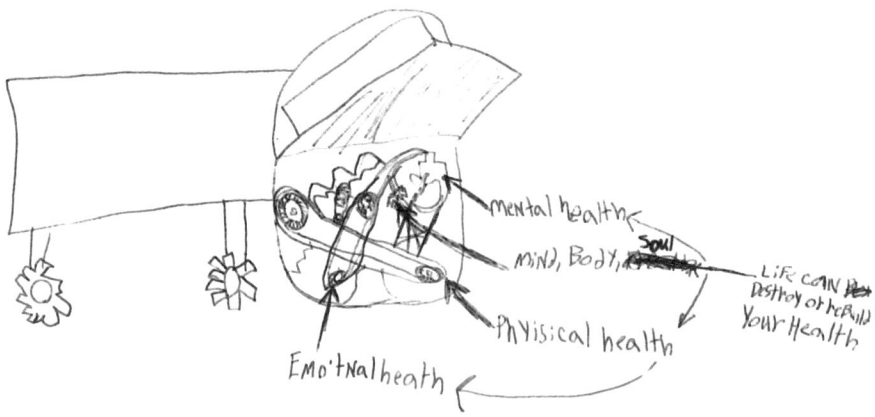

Fig. 3.6 Health is a car engine (step 1)

that part to make another thing work. Sometimes parts don't work and sometimes they do. It is just how you go through life with all your experiences and then eventually your car runs smoothly for a long period of time. And then you just kind of coast into death and then you are good.

Overall, participants drew a total of four houses, three cakes, two webs, two mazes, one car engine, one jenga game and several other unique ideas that included a candle and a beaker of water. We do not have room to report everyone's ideas, and yet all the children shared interesting insights into health through this activity. Once we had set up the task, the young people engaged with sustained creativity, interest and enthusiasm. Minimal prompts were required to keep conversation going. The rich, thick description that the children provided is another indication that the children were engaged and that the findings are credible.

Drawing Health Step 2: Adding the Research Base

One of our challenges in this activity was to use metaphors as a framework for talking about holistic health that allowed room for uniqueness, creativity and individual expression, but that also respected evidence-based thinking about health. We wondered if findings and recommendations from health research, shared in ways that were accessible to young people, could be incorporated into the children's metaphors in order to help them consider health evidence that is broader than their own personal ideas and experiences. Also, this was a way of introducing new ideas and information about health that may not have been previously known to the children. If demonstrated to be useful, this approach could address our concern about a potential disconnect between individualized attitudes and opinions about health and health behaviours, and the basic facts that some behaviours are well established as being poor health choices, while others can promote good health.

Our next step in our focus groups was to present the children with infographics and fact sheets that summarized evidence about health and its determinants. Our plan was to invite the children to consider their own drawings in light of this new information. The children could then decide if they wanted to develop or modify their drawings.

We introduced this exercise by stating "Here are some things that adults (including doctors and researchers) tell us are important to good health in people your age". We asked them to consider if anything they had seen in and/or learned from the infographics belonged in their picture, and if so, to incorporate it into their drawing. We gave them 15 min to think and draw, and then asked them to report on whether or how their picture (or metaphor) had evolved.

Application of Research to Individual Metaphors of Health

Overall, participants agreed that having an evidence base formed from research helped them to develop their ideas and think about their own health. Here are some of the things they told us:

> I got ideas from the graph about stuff to do to be healthy like the bike and I had not really thought about that. And also I read the graphs about how some people have a bad body image or they get bullied and how important self-confidence is for those people.

> [the research] made me think more about things like body image and confidence.

> I think [the research] helps you to know what the average person thinks or what the papers say about it because it may change your ideas and what you will draw next or what you might do differently.

One of the children told us that the type of infographic she was shown was "very familiar". She said "school shows these a lot" but they "don't let us read them. They just flash them for like two seconds and they are like, you should do this". For this child, connecting the information with her own picture was a very meaningful experience because "I have to think about it and think about what I am trying to get across and what it is trying to get across. I can relate it to the picture because now that I have thought about health and am connected to health". Another agreed. Applying the information to her own model of health was important because "this is my outlook on health. So it is easier to connect something to my outlook on health instead of a copy pasted image of health". The children were very clear: considering health information in an abstract way was nowhere near as meaningful as considering it in light of their own metaphors, their own health and their own experiences. This individualized and flexible approach allowed the children to engage with research *and* with their own health at one and the same time.

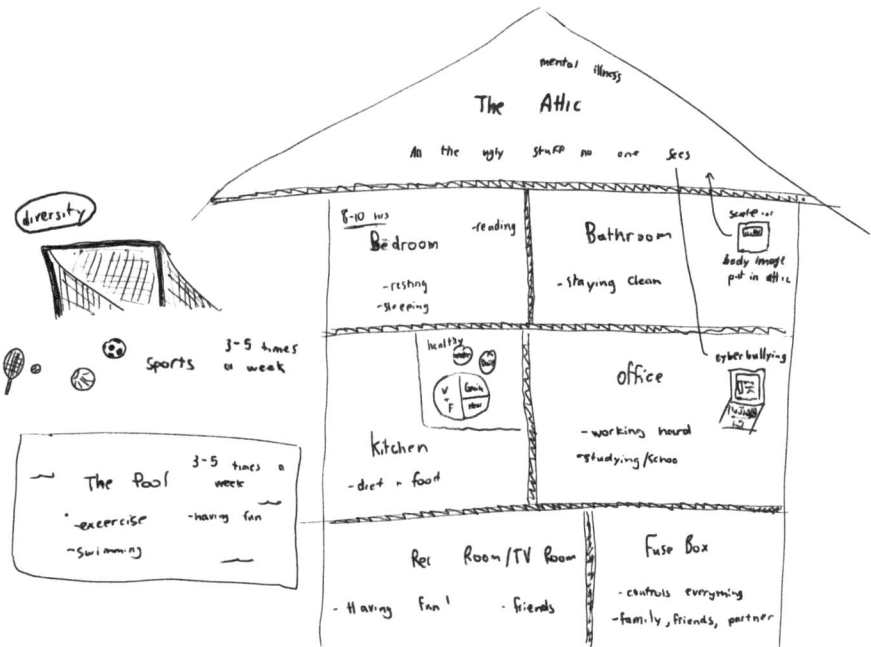

Fig. 3.7 Health is a house (step 2)

This first picture (Fig. 3.7) shows the changes our house artist made to her drawing after considering the research.

Here she describes her thought process as she developed her metaphor.

> I started adding specific things to my house. Before it was mostly happy things but then I started adding some of the bad things of health like I put a scale in the bathroom and how some people worry about their body image. And the things like cyber bullying and that kind of thing.

Another artist who drew a house made other adaptations:

> I added to my garage door that it is sleep…. Because it goes up and down all the time when cars are going in and out and that is kind of how your sleep is. So depending on how much work you have or how much after school stuff you have then your sleep varies. So it reminds me of a garage door opening and closing all the time. And then you know how there is the foundation stuff. I put that as some of the things about yourself like your body image and your self-consciousness so that if something happens to that kind of stuff then your whole house falls apart.

Figure 3.8 illustrates one way that her maze evolved after the child had considered the health evidence.

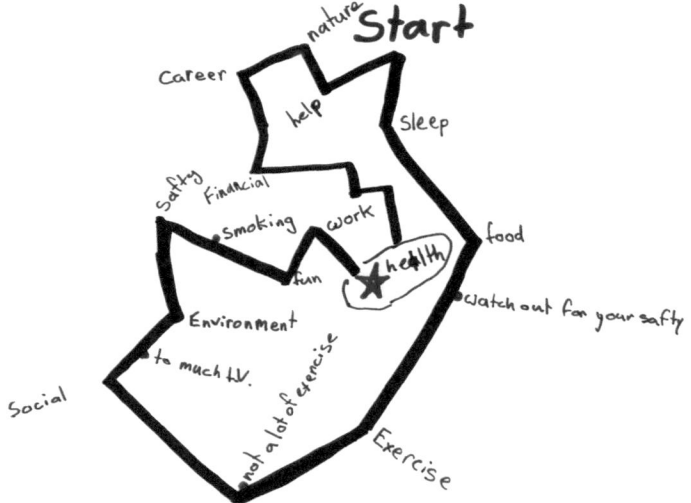

Fig. 3.8 Health is a maze (step 2)

The artist who had drawn this picture told us this:

> I changed my maze after I looked at some papers about health and I added more things like sleep or food because sometimes you have to go down a wrong turn to find out what was the right turn.

As the artist considered new ideas, her picture of a cake evolved as well (see Fig. 3.9).

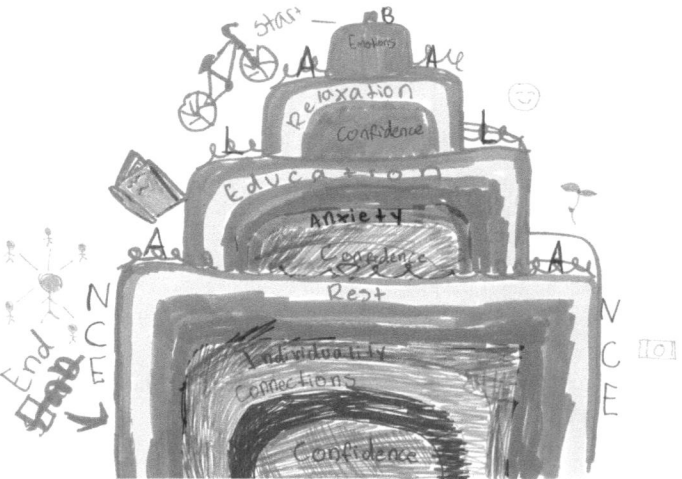

Fig. 3.9 Health is a cake (step 2)

Fig. 3.10 Health is a Jenga
game (step 2)

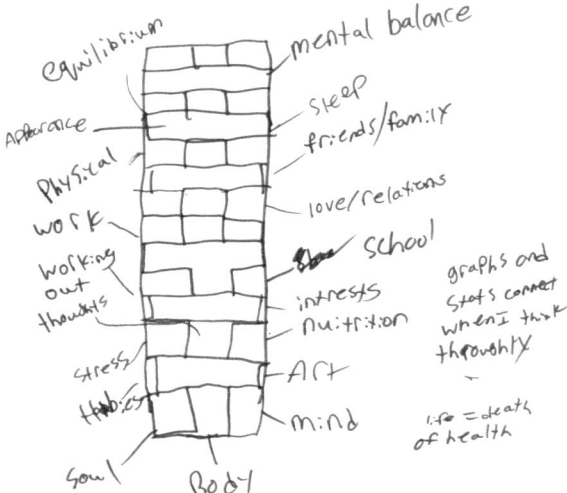

Here she describes what she did:

> I added stuff along the outside that affects your health, a bike for physical activity and a
> book for mental activity. I also added words that are important like rest and relaxation and
> education. I also added anxiety into the grey part. I put confidence in the center of all the
> layers because you have to have confidence in yourself to achieve all the good layers of the
> cake, like physical activity and perseverance to achieve your goals. The graphs about
> bullying gave me ideas about how important self-confidence is.

Finally, the Jenga artist developed his ideas as he considered new health information (Fig. 3.10).

> …to my Jenga at the bottom three blocks I added mind, body, and soul. Because they are
> the main things that hold up your health and I feel like school and life is that risky hand that
> always goes for the bottom blocks just to screw over the next person going for a block. And
> so it takes out some of the most important blocks because it has that power. Since it can
> change so many different things it can take out the major players in your health and just
> absolutely wreak havoc on you.

Reflection on the Introduction of This Research Base

One child told us that "if you just have health data but you don't have anything to
compare it against, or you can't apply it to your own life, then it is not worth as
much as if you can compare it against everything that has happened to you about
your own health". Her view was that looking at the infographics in isolation would
not be nearly as interesting as considering them as they relate to her own health and
life. Another child said "Obviously statistics are important because it is actual

research and it is facts. But we also need to draw on our own experiences and what we have been through". Respecting people's personal experience was vitally important to all of these children.

The order of the activities was also important. It appeared to have been important that the children established their own metaphors first, before they were given the infographics.

> I think if we had all started with [the infographics] then we would have all had the same information and a lot of our drawings would have looked the same or similar. And then it wouldn't have really been our health. I think when we started by doing our own drawings then we all picked what was important for us and that is important for each person to do. And we need to take time to consider…I mean this research is great but it is all about the average person and not the individual.

Interestingly, the children did not always agree with the infographic. One example related to reading. This girl read the infographic and reflected:

> On this graph it says for 2 to 3 times a week it says reading. And I feel like you should probably read more than 2 to 3 times a week for stretching your mind and to help your mental health…. I think most people should read more than 2 or 3 times a week. Some people it is harder for them to focus so they could listen to an audio book or something. And you could do that while exercising.

It was clear that the overarching flexibility of the metaphors was still important. One girl noted on her worksheet that "not all guidelines apply to everyone" and above these words she had sketched "different for everyone".

For all the participants, it appeared that introducing the research evidence base in the context of their own unique metaphors made their engagement with the research much more powerful. They took great care to creatively apply the research base to their own unique models of health.

Drawing Health Step 3: Holistic Conceptions of Health

We come full circle now and back to the concept of holism. Our primary goal was to observe if and how the use of metaphors could practically assist young people to think about health holistically. To do this, we encouraged the children to think about their metaphor as a whole picture of health rather than just focussing on the individual parts. We also gave each child a set of pictures to consider. Instead of more infographics, these pictures now reflected existing holistic models of health. They included the Indigenous medicine wheel, an ecological model of health designed for children, and a picture of the earth. We then asked the participants to consider whether or not these pictures helped them to think of something they wanted to add to their drawing or helped them to see their drawings differently.

Overall, the children reacted positively both to drawing metaphors to reflect their health and to the idea of holistic health. One said:

> I think… that it is more beneficial to look at health all at once and think about everything at the same time rather than focusing on sections. Like in school you said if we take health we would probably do a couple of classes on nutrition and a couple on safety and then some on exercise and that kind of thing. But we never really look at everything all at once, which I think would be the best way to do it.

As the children reflected on their metaphors holistically, many of them told us they started to see health differently. One child told us that from this exercise "I've learned and figured out a different perspective of health than I've had before". A girl reflected on what she learned through participating in the focus group and engaging with the various pictures and infographics, and hearing the ideas of the other children. She said:

> I find it interesting that there are so many aspects and categories to health. When I think health I think healthy food and exercise but they're so many different categories like spirituality, career, relationships …. I have learned that there are different ingredients to a healthy life other than the basic few. I also learned that the definition of health varies from one person to another.

As we asked the children to consider their health as a whole, new ideas continued to emerge. One boy who had been drawing a cake told us that, like a cake, health could even have a secret ingredient, "And it might be something that you know but no one else does. And it could be something that even you don't know about but it is still there".

The idea that came up most often, and most strongly, related to balance.

> One thing that I learned about is that I should work on having a balance on all of the parts of health because there are a lot more than I thought there was before.

> I learned how important balance of the parts is because I'd never really thought about it before. It gave me the idea to make sure I keep an equality in my life between my academic health and physical health and not have one better than the other. I should work on my physical more to balance it out.

The boy who had drawn the Jenga game told us that "balance is one of the main things of health for me because for good health you need to balance all the parts of health". He also told us that his

> ideas of health changed a lot because I realized the importance of every part of health. So with the Jenga box each and every block is important to the whole of health and that is what I learned. I also think that it is important to use holistically because it makes them realize the importance of everything and makes them live healthier lives because they can balance what they need and everything. Um three like I believe that the whole is bigger than the sum of the parts because the parts benefit each other to make each one stronger. So again if you put two parts together then it will make each other stronger.

Overall, by the end of this exercise, whether the children were using a cake, a house, a Jenga game or a car engine, many of them told us that they had formed new ideas about health or that their ideas about health had changed. The quality of metaphors themselves may partially explain this. As we pointed out in Chap. 2, when "this" is like "that", each conceptual category informs the other and new, alternative, and creative perspectives are formed. Certainly, this is what we saw in our study.

The second holistic idea reflected in our data relates to the interconnectedness of the different aspects of health. In particular, participants talked about what happens if one part of health (or ingredient, or Jenga block) is taken out, and how it would impact the whole:

> If you took rest and sleep out that would affect a lot of things. I forget where but it said that not having enough sleep will increase your stress and then you wouldn't want to do as many physical things and you would feel less motivated. And then your mental health would also start going downhill... It is like if one thing falls over then it will knock over a bunch of other things... So it is like a domino effect. If one thing is lacking then it will affect others.

Another child described these connections:

> Using my example of the Jenga blocks - if you just see a single block from the Jenga pile sitting on the table it kind of sucks honestly. You don't get excited by seeing a wooden block just sitting on a table. You would get excited by seeing the stack ready to play and friends around you and ready to play with you and stuff. So that kind of thing where your health is way better if you have all the pieces together because then it benefits you way more than it would if it was missing a few. And they all work together as well. So if you have good mental and body health that helps with all the other parts of that. Sometimes say your mental health if you are really into being fit that really helps with your physical health as well. So if you have more pieces then they work better with each other and it makes a bigger part than what they would be by themselves.
>
> So yeah.

We asked him if the other pieces would be impacted if he took out one piece.

> Totally. Like I said sometimes mental health can help with your physical health and vice versa. So if you take out part of your mental health then you will also lose some of your physical health as well. So different parts of your health can affect other parts of your health, meaning that even if it does not seem major at the time, taking one piece out of your health will diminish the rest of them by quite a bit. Yeah.

The interconnectedness of the many components of health made a real impression on our participants, regardless of the metaphor with which they had worked. One participant shared that her ideas about health had changed throughout our activity "because I realized the importance of every part of health.... The parts benefit each other making them stronger".

The new ideas or connections that the young people considered as a result of thinking about health as a holistic construct were not always sophisticated. Sometimes this new property was simply adding a new category of health to their drawing, and often the new connection was fairly basic. What was important was that the children were having the chance to have these realizations, and to make these connections for themselves. When children develop a holistic framework for thinking about health, they will be able to build on it as they develop cognitively, and they will be able to build on it throughout their life.

Holistic Health: Towards an Ecological Model

Most children stuck to drawing pictures about their immediate selves—their physical, mental, emotional, spiritual and social spheres of life. However, one of the older participants did something with her picture that we found intriguing. She started with a house, which can be seen in Fig. 3.1. She developed her house further as we discussed the research base. This can be seen in Fig. 3.7.

Towards the end of the focus group, she told us that health was much bigger than she realized, and shared some ideas. She said that working with the metaphor of a house "was interesting and it showed us that there are no parts of health that stand alone and they all connect." She had started by drawing a house, and by the end of the exercise, she had drawn a small city, complete with a bus route across the whole thing so that everything could connect, and told us that her picture was much bigger than she thought it was going to be when she started. Here it is in Fig. 3.11.

The child who drew this picture told us this:

Okay. So I started a new one and it is not 100% finished. I was doing a house and then I kind of figured that there were not enough things to put into a house so I turned it into a little city. And I have different places that represent different things. My house is in the middle and then a friend's house is beside it because it is important to have good friends and to be happy. So there are different sections like the doctor and the dentist to get

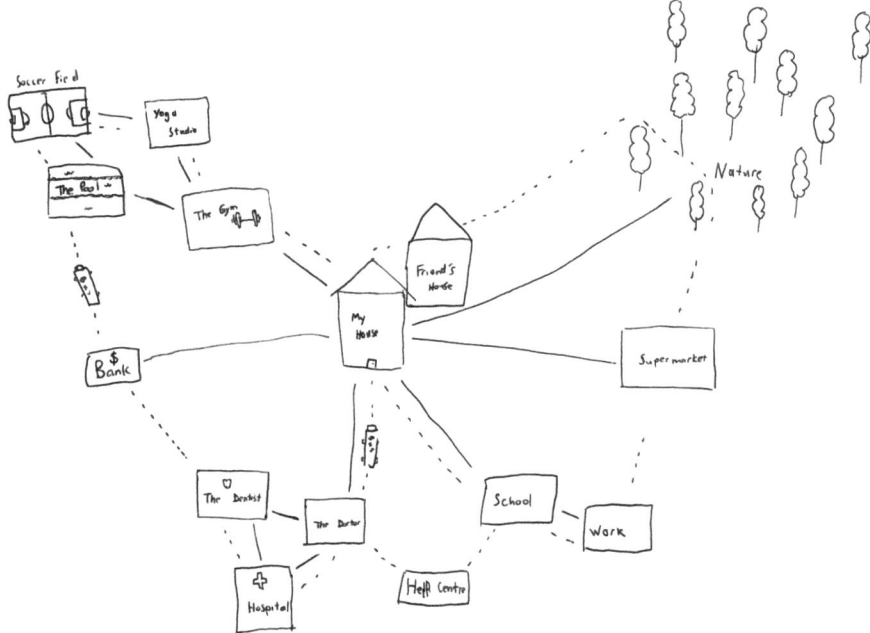

Fig. 3.11 Health is a house (step 3)

check-ups and stuff. There is the gym and the pool over here because that is important to me. There is a section here that kept saying spiritual health. My family is not very religious but that is important to a lot of people and I think we need to still embrace it. So I put a little yoga studio so it is Zen and stuff. And then…it said something about financial health. I don't many of us think of that much. We rely on our parents but I did put a little bank. There are different places that represent health.

With very little guidance, this child had developed the beginnings of a very good ecological model that described many determinants of health from her own viewpoint. She was invested in her pictures and her ideas, and concluded by telling us that working on her picture helped her think a lot more about how everything is connected all of the time. Her work is an illustrative example of how this kind of approach can be used to help children think about health in a variety of holistic ways.

A Strength and a Caution

The theme "different for everyone", which we saw reported so strongly in Chap. 2, continued to emerge clearly, right to the end of our study. One of the most poignant examples of this idea is reported here:

I think it is important to understand that health is different for everyone, especially kids our age since we are growing and stuff. In school when you learn about health they always tell you the things that you should do but they should be different for different kinds of people. So things like if they tell you, you need this much type of food. But you might have some condition where you can't eat that kind of food and so different things that apply differently to everyone…. there are always rigid guidelines to follow. And I think they need to be more flexible to be able to apply it to everyone.

The use of metaphors clearly facilitated the flexibility for which the children were looking.

There are many benefits to flexible models of health, and overall, this exercise was highly successful and resonated very well with the children. However, we do not recommend this activity without the second step, in which evidence-based health knowledge is introduced. Otherwise, we may well end up endorsing the idea that health is whatever a given person wants it to be. While there is value in customized, and even subjective approaches to health, we hope that we have demonstrated that there is also value in learning about how to better our health behaviours and practices by learning from the best available evidence.

When a healthy desire for customized approaches to health is balanced with a strong evidence base of health research, millennial children may reap the benefits of a model of health that is "different for everyone" but at the same time, is rooted in solid evidence. Likewise, a balanced approach will involve valuing young people's ideas, and yet challenging views that are in contradiction with scientifically established information about long-term consequences of poor health choices. If this is done, today's young people may reap the benefits of a model of health that is "different for everyone" but at the same time, rooted in knowledge and wisdom.

The theory of holism tells us that new ideas or properties emerge from the whole that are not present when solely looking at the individual parts, and further, that the parts are interdependent and gain new meaning in the context of the whole. Our findings from this small study suggest that metaphors can be powerful tools for facilitating this kind of holistic thinking about health.

The practical implications of these findings are many, and we will return to them again in Chap. 5. But first, we turn to quantitative methods, and explore their applicability to the theory of holism as it relates to child health.

Key Insights from This Chapter

- Metaphors are powerful tools (even "cognitive shortcuts") that help children think about abstract concepts in relation to concepts that are more familiar
- A customized approach to child health can have many strengths, but needs to be approached with caution, and be balanced with a base of research evidence

Key Findings

- We conducted a second qualitative study to explore the utility of using metaphors for engaging with children about holistic health

  - Along with the cake, the house, the web and the maze, two new metaphors were proposed by participants—a Jenga game and a car engine
  - Children found the metaphors to be both flexible and useful
  - Metaphors were a useful tool for helping children learn about health, and also to absorb and consider the information contained in evidence-based infographics
  - As participants reflected on their own metaphors, their ideas were in keeping with the properties important to holism: (1) New ideas, particularly around balance, emerged that were not present when studying the individual parts; and (2) The parts appeared to gain new meaning in relation to the whole

References

DiCarlo, M. A., Gibbons, J. L., Kaminsky, D. C., Wright, J. D., & Stiles, D. A. (2000). Street children's drawings: Windows into their life circumstances and aspirations. *International Social Work, 43,* 107–120.

Idler, E. L., & Benyamini, Y. (1997). Self-rated health and mortality: A review of twenty-seven community studies. *Journal of Health and Social Behavior, 38*(1), 21–37.

Merriman, B., & Guerin, S. (2006). Using children's drawings as data in child-centred research. *The Irish Journal of Psychology, 27*(1–2), 48–57.

Michaelson, V., Pickett, W., Vandemeer, E., Taylor, B., & Davison, C. (2016). A mixed methods study of Canadian adolescents' perceptions of health. *International Journal of Qualitative Studies on Health and Well-being, 11*(1), 32891.

Onyango-Ouma, W., Aagaard-Hansen, J., & Jensen, B. B. (2004). Changing concepts of health and illness among children of primary school age in Western Kenya. *Health Education Research, 19*(3), 326–339.

Piko, B. F., & Bak, J. (2006). Children's perceptions of health and illness: Images and lay concepts in preadolescence. *Health Education Research, 21*(5), 643–653.

Pridmore, P., & Bendelow, G. (1995). Images of health: Exploring beliefs of children using the 'draw-and-write' technique. *Health Education Journal, 54*(4), 473–488.

Psych, C., & Larsen, J. E. (2004). "I am a puzzle": Adolescence as reflected in self-metaphors. *Canadian Journal of Counselling, 38*(4), 246.

Shaffer, D., Fisher, P., Lucas, C. P., Dulcan, M. K., & Schwab-Stone, M. E. (2000). NIMH diagnostic interview schedule for children version IV (NIMH DISC-IV): Description, differences from previous versions, and reliability of some common diagnoses. *Journal of the American Academy of Child and Adolescent Psychiatry, 39*(1), 28–38.

Thomas, G. V., & Jolley, R. P. (1998). Drawing conclusions: A re-examination of empirical and conceptual bases for psychological evaluation of children from their drawings. *British Journal of Clinical Psychology, 37,* 127–139.

Chapter 4
Testing the Theory of Holism in Child Health Settings Using Quantitative Approaches

Organic or unified 'wholes' have value and qualities which are inherently different from, and cannot be reduced to, the sum of their individual parts.

—Christakis

Abstract In this chapter we present the findings of research that employed quantitative methods. We did this in order to illustrate that it is possible to conduct empirical studies of holistic concepts in the field of child health. Four examples of holistic assessment are presented, representing development of: (1) A composite measure describing contextual determinants of health (family systems); (2) A composite measure describing engagement in multiple risk-taking; and (3) A composite measure of self-perceived child health status; and confirmation of (4) A single item measure of self-perceived child health status. All analyses used data from the 2014 Canadian Health Behaviour in School-aged Children (HBSC) study, a sample comprised of 29,784 grade 6–10 students from 377 schools across Canada. Overall, we demonstrate that not only is it possible to create holistic measures by applying quantitative methods, but that these measures are also stronger predictors/correlates of health than their individual components. The individual components are interrelated and their health-related risks are interdependent. Finally, the single self-rated health item is briefly described as a simple, yet potentially useful and powerful measure of holistic health.

Keywords Epidemiology · Quantitative methods · Factor analysis · Paediatrics · Determinants of health

We now turn to quantitative research methods, which offer a complementary approach to our study of the concept of holism and its application to child health. Quantitative methods can be used to summarize important health trends and patterns, and to quantify attitudes, opinions, behaviours, health status and other defined variables. This is important, because quantitative samples are generally much larger

© The Author(s) 2018
V. Michaelson et al., *Holistic Health in Children: Conceptualization, Assessment and Potential*, SpringerBriefs in Well-Being and Quality of Life Research, DOI 10.1007/978-3-319-64831-6_4

and more representative than qualitative samples, making the findings more generalizable to a large population. Thus, they complement the richness, depth and insights gleaned from our qualitative enquiry. We use these methods to help us move beyond a theoretical discussion of holism or how it is experienced (qualitative) in order to develop ways to apply this theory to the assessment of health and its determinants in child populations (quantitative).

We offer four examples of quantitative analyses. In the epidemiological tradition, each example represents an attempt to measure some aspect of child health in composite. Our first analysis focuses on one important set of determinants of health: the qualities of families and family systems and how they relate to health indicators among youth, including self-perceived positive health status. The second focuses on the assessment of risk-taking behaviours in populations of young people and the influence of these behaviours on their health. The third explores the health status of young people as a latent construct (a theoretical construct that cannot be observed directly and thus cannot be measured directly), and whether it is indeed possible to assess its various domains as a unified whole. And the fourth explores a very simple one-question self-rated health item. These analyses are meant to be illustrative and not exhaustive. Collectively, they point to the potential for aspects of health to be considered as systems, the complexity of which can be viewed and measured as holistic constructs that have meaning and value.

Our Quantitative Research Opportunity

Data for each of these four quantitative analyses come from the 2014 *Health Behaviour in School-aged Children* study, or "HBSC" (Currie, Gabhainn, Godeau, & International HBSC Network Coordinating Committee, 2009; Freeman, King, & Pickett, 2015). The HBSC study is one of the largest health promotion surveys of children in the world, and is affiliated with the World Health Organization (WHO). It aims to increase understanding of health and its determinants in populations of young people. Each of the authors of this book is a Canadian investigator in the HBSC study, and Dr. Pickett has participated in the conduct of this survey in Canada since 1996.

The 2014 version of the HBSC survey chronicled the experiences of some 29,784 young people from 377 schools across Canada. Participants were in grades 6 to 10, and while we refer to them as children throughout this chapter, we are mainly referring to children in the preadolescent and adolescent age range of 11–15 years. This rich source of data provided the opportunity to test the theory of holism from four different perspectives. For interested readers, a more detailed description of the HBSC survey methods can be found in Appendix C.

Example 1: Analysing Family Systems Through a Holistic Measure

Characteristics of families are among the strongest and most consistent influences on the overall health of young people. For most, they provide basic essentials of life and an environment that fosters early childhood development (Bronfenbrenner, 1986). Families come in a diversity of configurations, and family systems in contemporary societies tend to be varied and complex. However, there may be holistic qualities of families that transcend these complexities and could be captured in a composite measure. Some family qualities may reflect possible harmful environments for growing children, and others may be protective. Through this analysis, our goal was to explore these ideas, and develop a composite measure that permitted analysis and some reflection on the theory of holism.

We put together our composite measure using data from the 2014 Canadian HBSC study (Freeman, King, & Pickett, 2015). Methodologically, we drew on lessons from UNICEF's Report Card series (Adamson, 2010). The United Nations Children's Fund (UNICEF) is a non-profit organization that works to ensure the well-being of children globally. UNICEF's scientific arm, the UNICEF Innocenti Research Centre, is most famously known for its production of several "Report Cards" describing the health of children across countries and cultures. The authors of the UNICEF Report Card series have in fact long experimented with the development of composite measures of health as applied to children and their social environments. In Report Card 9: *The Children Left Behind*, they created a composite measure of child well-being (Adamson, 2010). By combining multiple items that captured different aspects of well-being this composite measure provided a more holistic approach to assessment of child well-being than examining the individual measures on their own. This measure focused on the socio-economic conditions that surrounded young people, and was subsequently used to identify how far behind their peers the most disadvantaged children were being allowed to fall.

While the results of UNICEF Report Card 9 confirmed the presence of profound inequalities in child well-being in some of the world's wealthiest countries, the long-term contributions of this report card may in fact be methodological. We adapted UNICEF's methodological approach to the development of different composite measures, including holistic assessment of "family systems". Following the UNICEF precedent, we first selected a range of eleven indicators that described specific components of family systems (Appendix C). In choosing the indicators we were limited by two factors: the indicator had to have been (1) measured in the 2014 HBSC survey, and; (2) measured on a continuous scale (in order to apply the UNICEF method) (Adamson, 2010). As our focus was on capturing the family system as an important determinant of health, a priori it was decided to only consider family characteristics that could, at least theoretically, impact the health and well-being of young people.

Next, using individual observations from students that participated in the 2014 Canadian HBSC study, we conducted an exploratory factor analysis (Suhr, 2006) with the eleven indicators. Exploratory factor analysis is a statistical method commonly used to develop measures or scales for constructs that are not directly observable. Based on conventional psychometrics (high Cronbach's alpha values; acceptable fit statistics from confirmatory factor analyses), this analysis suggested the importance of four different items that contributed to a larger scale or measure. Again, a more thorough description of these methods can be found in Appendix C. The four items described family material wealth, family support, family meal practices, and family neighbourhood social capital (Fig. 4.1). Following the UNICEF method, we then standardized each of the four indicators to a common scale with a mean of 100 and standard deviation of 10, and combined them into a composite, holistic family systems scale by averaging their values.

Using our new composite measure of family systems, we were able to assign a holistic family systems score to each of the youth who participated in the 2014 Canadian HBSC study. For the subsequent analyses, we divided the youth based on their family systems score into five equal groups (quintiles), from the least to highest functioning families. We then examined the proportion of students in each of these groups reporting a variety of health indicators in a series of descriptive analyses. Our findings appeared to tell a strong and consistent story: as family system scores got larger (indicative of better functioning families), so too did the proportion of young people reporting positive indications of health.

For example, where we examined various indicators of child health (Fig. 4.2), this positive relationship was reflected in reports of young people's self-perceived health status, life satisfaction (measured using a standard measure called the "Cantril ladder") (Cantril, 1965), peer support (using an existing HBSC scale), and psychosomatic symptoms (a scale that included headache, stomach ache, back ache, feeling low, irritability or bad temper, feeling nervous, difficulties in getting to sleep, feeling dizzy) (Hetland, Torsheim, & Aarø, 2002). In fact, this same trend was true for virtually every health outcome that we examined, whether that was

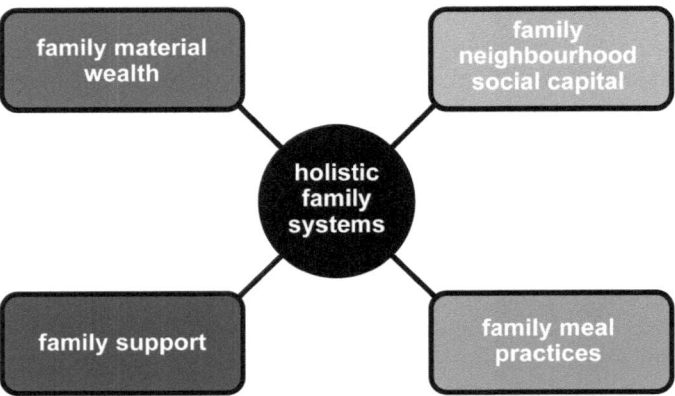

Fig. 4.1 Schematic diagram illustrating the factor analytically derived items that constitute a composite measure of holistic family systems, HBSC Canada, 2014

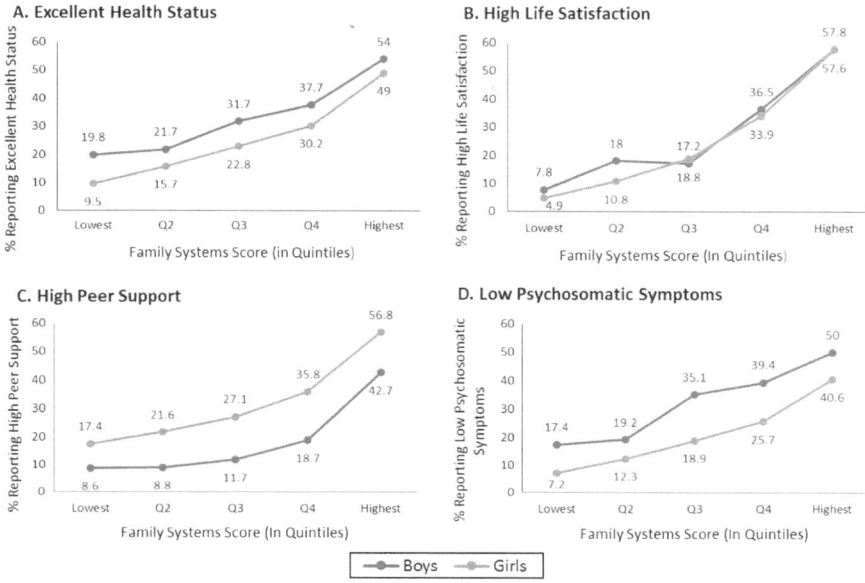

Fig. 4.2 Proportion of children reporting positive health indicators by quintile of family systems score and gender, HBSC Canada, 2014

health behaviours (e.g., reductions in child risk-taking behaviours), emotional health, or social health outcomes (Michaelson, Pickett, King, & Davison, 2016).

Even more pertinent for our study of holism, in virtually all of the comparisons that were made, the holistic family systems measure was more predictive of child health status than were the individual components that made up this scale. To illustrate, in Fig. 4.3 we can see that the holistic family systems measure is a much stronger predictor of excellent health status in children than the independent effects of any one of its individual components, comparing the highest (or most well-off) group with the lowest (or least well-off).

Using the same regression approach we also considered the interrelatedness of the individual components by examining whether there were any significant interaction effects. While a number of the interactions were "borderline" in terms of statistical significance, one in particular stood out. The positive impact of high family support on excellent health status was much greater in children from the least well-off families (RR = 3.32 (95% CI: 2.20–5.01) than in children from the most well-off families (RR = 1.71 (95% CI: 1.49–1.96), illustrating the interdependence of these two family characteristics. In other words, family support seems to be more important to the health of youth from less affluent families.

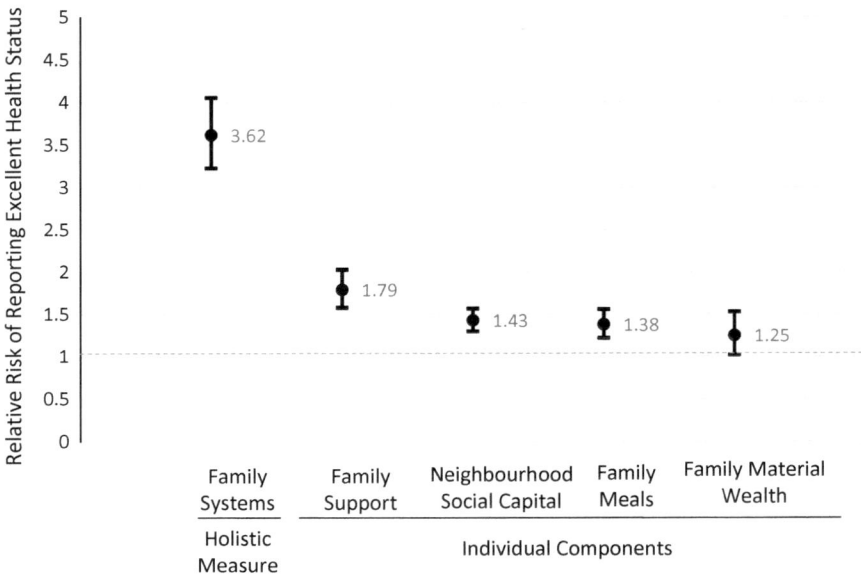

Fig. 4.3 Relative Risk (RR) of reporting excellent self-rated health status, comparing the highest (most functional family systems) versus the lowest (least functional) groups defined by quintile; HBSC Canada, 2014. The bars represent a 95% confidence interval

How Does This Analysis Reflect Holistic Thinking?

The framework we have used to guide our work on holistic health suggests that if something is holistic, it has at least two distinct properties. First, there is some kind of emergent property in the whole that is not reflected by the component parts. In the above modeling, while there is not a new or different emergent property per se, what we did observe was a consistent strengthening of the pattern that was reflective of the multiplicative natures of risks and protections. By combining the component parts into a single composite (holistic) measure, we created a more stable and reliable predictor of health than when the individual components were considered on their own.

The second core property relates to the interconnectedness of the parts—the idea that the parts cannot be fully understood if they are isolated from the whole. When we looked at the component parts that went into this composite measure, we learned that there are some over-riding qualities of families that influence health, and the individual components provide the mechanisms by which that occurs. We discovered that the health risks associated with an individual component may not be accurately or fully captured if the other related components are not also considered. In other words, the components can interact to produce varying levels of health so that the risk associated with one component depends on the presence or absence of another component. In our example we showed that family support had a differential impact on the child's health depending on the level of affluence of the child's family.

This analysis demonstrates the value in examining the properties of complex systems, such as families, holistically instead of by a more reductionist approach that relies on individual indicators of family function. By considering multiple family characteristics simultaneously, one is better able to predict the impact of that set of health determinants (characteristics of families), on a child's health. In reality, multiple characteristics of families are not found in isolation, but rather they exist as part of a system and collectively come together to impact on the health of the young person.

Example 2: Analysis of Child Risk-taking Through a Holistic Measure

We then turned to another domain of children's lives, engagement in risk-taking and problem behaviours, in order to determine whether or not holistic thinking in this context has practical value.

In the early 1990s, a US-based social researcher named Dr. Ron Jessor developed a concept that he termed "problem behaviour theory" (Jessor, 1991). Amongst his many foundational ideas, Jessor contended that young people often engage in risk-taking behaviours that are more typical of adults as one means of transitioning socially to adulthood. He observed that risk-taking is actually experimental and transitory in many young people during this critical period of development. However, other times, when such behaviours become normative and cluster together, this is potentially indicative of the beginnings of a high-risk lifestyle that is detrimental to health.

In his research, Jessor (1991) examined these groups of young people who tended to engage in many different forms of risk behaviour simultaneously. This clustered risk-taking was of particular concern. According to his research, the specific risk-taking behaviour—whether it was smoking, alcohol or other drug misuse, truancy, or unprotected sex—was not that consequential. Rather, it was the influence of engaging in multiple risk-taking in some children that was most associated with negative health trajectories and outcomes.

Although negative in terms of its influence on health, there was something holistic in this idea. In other words, there is something about the coming together of multiple risks in composite that is profound, and poses hazards to the child beyond the individual constituent risks. Jessor's ideas were novel at the time. Traditionally, child studies of risk-taking had considered the independent effects of behaviours expressed in isolation. Using our holistic lens, we therefore decided to consider child risk-taking in a more composite sense as Jessor did, and explore whether this holistic lens provided additional insight into the origins of child health.

The 2014 HBSC survey contains a number of questions on risk-taking behaviours, many of which mirror the list that Jessor originally considered (Jessor, 1991). We reviewed the HBSC questionnaire for all possible related questions, and selected 22 of them that were asked to Grade 6–8 students. Among others these included lifetime smoking history, use of alternative tobacco products, frequency of alcohol consumption, lifetime drunkenness history, bullying others, physical fighting, and energy drink consumption.

By examining frequency distributions, we could classify each behaviour reported by young people into "high risk" (extensive), "medium risk" (moderate) or "low risk" (minimal) categories of engagement (Table 4.1). The available HBSC sample was randomly split into two, and an exploratory factor analysis for categorical variables was conducted on one half, and then confirmed in the other (refer to Appendix C for more detail on methods) (Suhr, 2006). This exploratory factor analysis was used to examine which subset of behaviours was strongly related to a common underlying construct, or 'factor'. From the 22 risk-taking behaviours considered, three unique factors were identified (Kwong, Klinger, Janssen, & Pickett, 2015). One of these was 'Overt Risk-taking', which included the seven behaviours previously described.

A composite scale was created by summing reports for each of the variables together, using weights that were obtained from the exploratory factor analysis. The behaviours that related most strongly to the underlying construct were given greater weight and thus contributed more to the overall score. Relative weights for each behaviour included in the composite scale are represented visually within the word cloud below (Fig. 4.4). For example, lifetime smoking history has a greater contribution to a young person's overt risk-taking score than their energy drink consumption. Through the factor analyses the composite scale was found to be valid and internally reliable (Kwong et al., 2015).

Table 4.1 Category definitions for risk behaviours included in the composite over risk-taking scale, grade 6–8 students, HBSC Canada, 2014

Risk behaviours	Low risk	Medium risk	High risk
Number of days they smoked cigarettes in their life	Never	1–29 days	30+ days
Alternative tobacco products (e.g., e-cigarette, flavoured tobacco…)	Never used any	Used one once or more	Used several once or more
Frequency of alcohol consumption (e.g., beer, wine, cider, liquor/spirits…)	Never drank any	Rarely	Every month-Every day
Number of times they got drunk in their life	Never	Once	2+ times
Number of times they got into a physical fight in the last year	No fights	Once	2+ times
Frequency of personal bullying behaviour on others	No bullying	Once-3 times a month	Once a week or more
Frequency of energy drink consumption in a typical week	Never	Less than or once a week	2–4 times a week or more

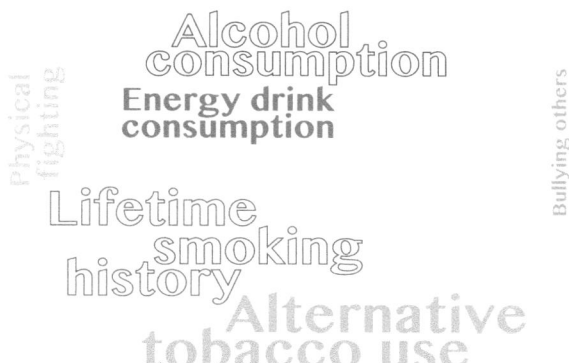

Fig. 4.4 An illustrative example of the overt risk behaviours used is found in this second holistic model. Font size is reflective of the relative impact of the behaviour on the overall latent construct

The next step was to correlate reports of individual risk-taking behaviours made by the students to a variety of self-reported health outcomes. We started with an outcome of different types of injuries (e.g., school and fighting injuries), one of the most common and important acute health outcomes experienced by Canadian children. What we observed was somewhat predictable from Jessor's theory. Engagement in each of the seven different risk behaviours elevated the risk for reporting the occurrence of different types of injury, but by a small increment. Yet clearly, engagement in risk-taking was associated with the occurrence of injury.

However, when the different risk behaviours were compiled together into a composite holistic measure, a more interesting pattern emerged (Fig. 4.5). As the

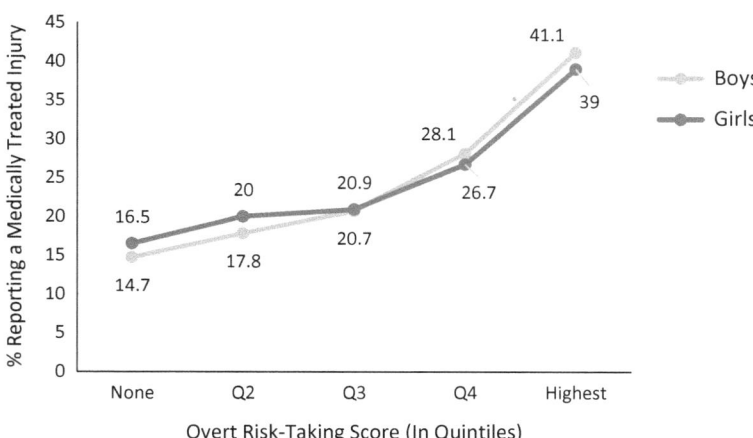

Fig. 4.5 Proportion of children in grade 6–8 reporting a medically treated non sport-related injury by quintiles of the holistic, overt risk-taking score, HBSC Canada, 2014

holistic score that summarized children's risk-taking went up, so did the occurrence of injury, but in a strong and multiplicative fashion. This was true for boys and girls and for every different type of injury reported. It also remained true after mathematical adjustment for variables that could confound this relationship. Observed risks were striking in their consistency. There was something in this composite holistic score that was capturing a phenomenon that far exceeded the effects of its individual components, at least in terms of one common health outcome. When multiple risk-taking behaviours were considered in composite, or through a more holistic lens, they were a much stronger predictor of injury than when the individual risk-behaviours were considered on their own. A holistic assessment approach indeed was helpful.

We then extended this enquiry to consideration of other health outcomes, including psychosomatic symptoms and self-perceived health status. The latter is a particularly important indicator as, in addition to being a holistic concept, self-perceived health status during early stages of life is known to be predictive of health outcomes in adulthood. Young people who rate their health favourably are at lower risk of chronic disease outcomes and even premature mortality later in life (DeSalvo, Bloser, Reynolds, He, & Muntner, 2006; Kaplan et al., 1996).

As Fig. 4.6 shows, there was a strong relationship between higher scores on the holistic measure of child risk-taking and lower percentages of self-rated "excellent" health status. This was a particularly strong finding among girls. These findings were replicated nearly exactly when psychosomatic health was examined as the outcome.

Through further analyses of potential interactions, we also examined whether or not risks for injury associated with one behaviour differed in the presence or absence of another. For example, fighting was consistently associated with an

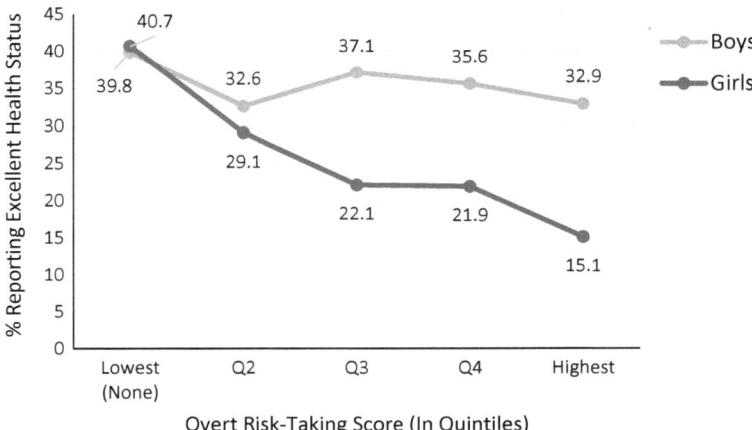

Fig. 4.6 Proportion of children in grade 6 to 8 reporting excellent health status by quintiles of the holistic, overt risk-taking score, HBSC Canada, 2014

increased risk for injury, but the risk was greater in youth who regularly consumed alcohol relative to those who abstained. This provided evidence of the inter-relatedness of these constituent parts that eventually were combined into the more holistic composite measure.

How Does This Analysis Reflect Holistic Thinking?

Using standard epidemiological analyses, we were able to demonstrate quantitatively that a composite risk-taking score was associated strongly and consistently with a variety of different health outcomes. As we observed in our first example, the size of observed effects was much stronger than would be predicted by the effects of the individual components. While we could not necessarily say that new properties emerged, there was a consistent strengthening of the pattern. For example, after adjusting for age, sex, socioeconomic status, and the six other overt risk-taking behaviours, youth in the high risk alcohol consumption group (approximately 15% of children surveyed) were 1.36 times (95% CI: 1.13 to 1.64) more likely to report a medically treated non sport-related injury than youth in the low risk group. In comparison, when using the holistic overt risk-taking scale, youth in the highest quintile (20% of children surveyed) were 2.63 (95% CI: 1.71 to 2.28) times more likely to report an injury than youth in the low risk group.

Child risk-taking therefore represented a second context related to child health for which the theory of holism appeared to hold. There is clearly an important and interdependent connection between the parts and moreover, the negative effects of each individual risk behaviour (or part) are most fully understood when viewed in relation to the whole.

Example 3: Creating a Holistic Measure for the Assessment of Child Health Status

Our third foray into applying quantitative methods to the study of holism and child health was concerned with developing a holistic measure of child health status. Our hope was to create a composite measure that incorporated the four domains of health as defined by the World Health Organization (WHO): physical, mental/emotional, social, and spiritual (WHO, 1948). According to the WHO, each of these domains of health must be satisfied in order to achieve optimal levels of health.

To create our measure of holistic health we first identified all of the continuous measures in the 2014 HBSC survey that assessed one of the four domains of health. In total there were ten different measures available for analysis (Appendix C). Then, just as we did in our previous analyses, we split the HBSC sample in half and using the first half, included all ten measures in an initial exploratory factor analysis.

Because our goal was to create a single composite measure, we forced a one factor solution, which we labelled as 'holistic health'. If a single factor had not been specified then we likely would have ended up with the ten measures grouping together into multiple factors representing each of the separate domains of health.

Using the WHO definition of health as a guide, we considered each of the four domains of health as equally important. Therefore we decided a priori to include a single measure, and only a single measure, representing each domain in the final scale. Based on factor loadings generated from the exploratory factor analysis, which quantify how strongly the variable is related to the underlying latent construct, measures with the weakest loadings were sequentially removed until only a single measure representing each domain remained (Fig. 4.7).

The UNICEF Report Card approach (Adamson, 2010) again provided us with a standardized method of combining measures from each of the domains into a single composite (holistic) measure. Once selected, each of the four measures was standardized onto a common scale with a mean of 100 and standard deviation of 10, and combined by averaging their values. The final holistic measure was inclusive of each of the four domains of health, and was essentially a "scale of scales" with higher scores indicative of better overall health, and lower scores indicating worse overall health. A confirmatory factor analysis, conducted on the second half of the sample, indicated acceptable model fit.

To examine how well this new measure captured the overall health status of children, we explored its construct validity (the degree to which the measure is measuring what it is intended to measure). We did this by first categorizing youth who participated in the 2014 HBSC study into five equal groups (quintiles) from least to most healthy based on their holistic health score. We then examined the proportion of children in each group that reported various health outcomes not included in the composite scale. We expected to see that the proportion reporting the outcome would increase across the quintiles for positive health outcomes, and

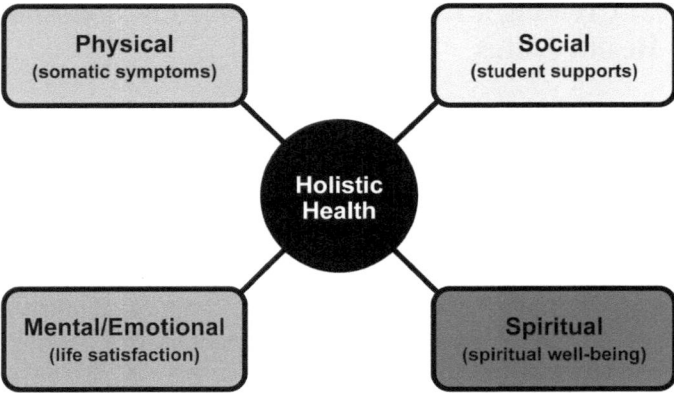

Fig. 4.7 Key domains that contribute to the composite measure used to describe the overall health of an individual, holistically

would decrease for negative ones. And if the theory of holism was reflected in this measure, these relationships would be much stronger and more consistent than if we substituted the individual components for the holistic scale.

This is exactly what we observed. The holistic health measure correlated strongly and consistently in the expected direction with all health indicators examined, including measures of diet, physical activity, sedentary behaviour, violence, and emotional health. Strong dose-response relationships were seen across the board. Further, the associations between the holistic measure and various health indicators were stronger and more consistent in terms of dose-response than the correlations between its individual components and the same health indicators.

Figure 4.8 provides an illustration of one such analysis, again revisiting self-perceived excellent health status as a focused outcome. For both boys and girls, one can see a graded, consistent and strong dose-related increase in the proportion of young people reporting excellent health as the holistic health score increases across the quintiles.

In additional analyses, we considered how the four domains included in the holistic measure interacted to predict excellent health status. Not surprisingly, the greater number of domains that children report as relatively high (in the top half compared to their peers), the greater their likelihood of having excellent health status; 54% of boys and 49% of girls who were high in all four domains compared to 39% and 32% who were high in three, and 29 and 21% who were high in only two (Fig. 4.9).

Acknowledging that optimal health is achieved when all four domains are high, we also examined whether being high in three domains of health could compensate for being low in the fourth. First, as expected we found that for every domain a greater proportion of youth who reported the domain as high reported excellent health status versus those who reported the domains as low (14–26% higher). We

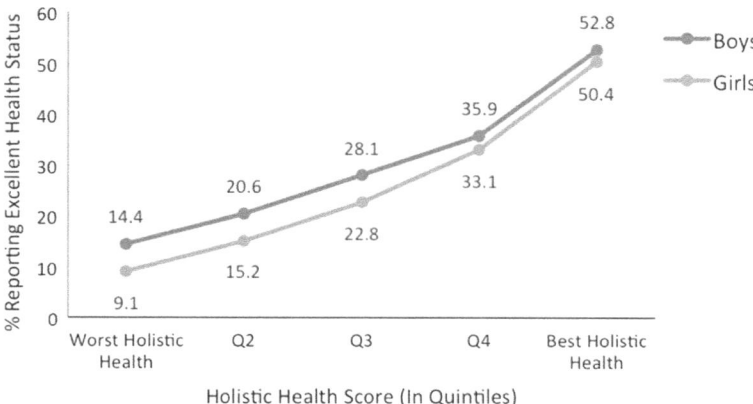

Fig. 4.8 Proportion of children reporting excellent health status by quintiles of the holistic health score, HBSC Canada, 2014

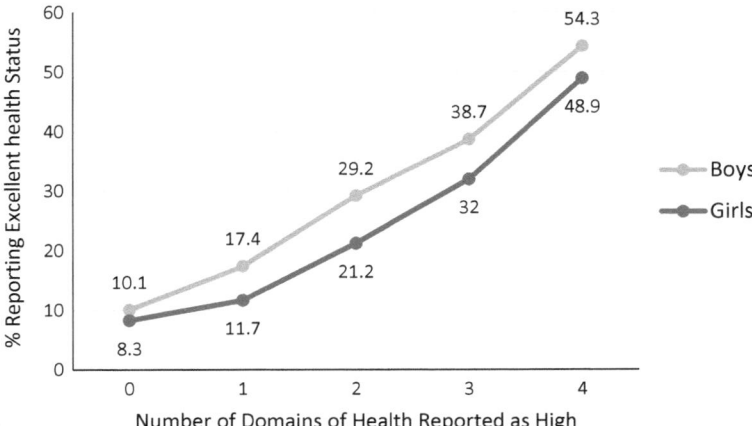

Fig. 4.9 Proportion of children reporting excellent health status by the number of domains of health (physical, mental/emotional, social, and spiritual) they reported as high (in the top half of children surveyed), HBSC Canada, 2014

then compared youth who reported the domain as high to the narrower subgroup of youth who were low in that domain, but high in the other three. For the domains of physical, social, and spiritual health the difference in the proportion with excellent health status either disappeared or reversed, suggesting that being high in three domains compensates for being low in the fourth. A similar pattern was seen for mental health, although not as strong. Reporting a high score in the other three domains of health did not fully compensate for having low mental health.

How Does This Analysis Reflect Holistic Thinking?

Similar to our previous examples, we have demonstrated that the holistic health measure is a stronger measure of health status than the individual components in terms of its association with various health indicators. It appears that the holistic measure is able to more accurately classify children according to their overall health status. Further, the findings suggest that when considered on their own, the separate domains of health may not give a true or full representation of an individual's health status. Optimal health appears to be achieved when all four domains of health are satisfied. Examining the individual domains on their own may not capture the larger, more informative picture of child health. For example, a child might have above average physical health, but in fact might be doing quite poorly overall. We also show that the separate domains of health are interrelated in that doing poorly in one domain can be overcome by doing well in the others. These findings further demonstrate the importance of holistic approaches to the assessment of child health.

Example 4: Self-rated Health

Throughout this chapter we considered self-rated health as an indicator of children's health status. Previous research tells us that the outcome of "self-rated health" is a powerful, single item measure that captures a holistic view of health among child populations (Joffer, Jerdén, Öhman, & Flacking, 2016). Children's responses to this seemingly simple question correlate to the physical, social, and mental aspects of their health. Quantitatively, this was observed in our study, as the single item measure of self-rated health correlated strongly with our composite measure of holistic health derived in the third example (Fig. 4.8). When youth are asked qualitatively how they interpret this question, again the multiple domains of health come out in their answers. It is a powerful measure because, on its own, it is prognostic of many long-term health outcomes including those associated with chronic disease, mental health status, and mortality (DeSalvo et al., 2006; Kaplan et al., 1996).

It remains unknown why this single item measure of health is such a powerful predictor of future health outcomes. One possible explanation is because of its flexibility. In our qualitative study, youth stressed the importance of allowing room for health to be different for everyone. It may be that for this very subjective measure the individual is able to interpret health in a way that is most meaningful to him or her. Children can define health according to their own perceptions and feelings, and this subjective measure allows them to adapt and capture what they perceive to be most important. Further, our quantitative findings suggest that this single item may actually be an efficient way of assessing the construct of holistic health. Its predictive power likely relates to the fact that it appears to be capturing this construct.

Conclusion: How Do All of These Analyses Reflect Holistic Thinking?

In this chapter, we set out to complement our theoretical discussion and qualitative findings by using quantitative research methods to apply basic principles of holism to aspects of the health of children. We hypothesized that revisiting holistic theories would provide new insights that could inform many aspects of children's health, and focused on assessment and measurement, and the contexts that possibly determine child health. Using established theory and established analytical approaches, we developed new holistic measures to describe family contexts, child risk-taking, and the health of young people in composite.

What was novel in these analyses was not a demonstration of the importance of these topics for the health of young people per se (that has already been well established in the literature), but rather the confirmation of the possibility and value of measuring complex aspects of health and its determinants holistically.

In each of our four examples, we argue that indeed, new properties emerge with the whole that are not clearly evidenced in the individual components that contribute to the whole. We see this mainly reflected not by an entirely new concept, but by the strength and consistency of the relationships observed, and their clarity compared to individual-based analyses. When determinants of health are examined in composite, we are better equipped to more accurately predict risk for poor outcomes in youth.

Further, in each of our first three examples, we observed that when the individual parts are isolated from the whole, we can miss important insights. Take for example our second analytical approach related to multiple risk behaviours. While looking at each behaviour on its own certainly has value, if that is the only approach that is taken, the cumulative effects are missed. The likely trajectory around the misuse of alcohol for someone who participates in this single risk behaviour is not the same as it is for another child who participates in multiple risk behaviours. And in our third analytical example, we see the interdependence of the four domains of health. For example, someone with low physical health but high spiritual, mental and social health could still report having excellent health status. Low physical health in a child who reports positive health in the other three domains is again, reflective of a very different whole person health experience. Clearly, the interactions between the four domains are important. As Christakis (2012) suggests, a unified whole cannot be reduced to the sum of its individual parts, and something is potentially happening related to health outcomes that cannot be fully understood by looking at individual components alone.

Holistic measurement has the potential to provide new insights that can inform etiological and preventive research. Our findings in these analyses confirm that potentially new, different, or stronger properties emerge when systems are studied as a whole, and further, that the individual parts are understood more fully when viewed in the context of the whole. This is in keeping with longstanding philosophies and models of health.

Our next—and final—chapter is integrative. We bring together what we have learned through qualitative and quantitative methods, and offer practical recommendations related to children's health.

Key Insights from This Chapter

- Holistic constructs can be quantified, and it is possible to create valid and reliable holistic (composite) measures of health and its determinants
- Holistic approaches to quantitative analysis can increase our understanding of determinants of health

Key Findings

- We conducted four examples of quantitative analyses to measure some aspect of child health in composite

- Compared to the individual components, holistic measures are stronger, and more consistent predictors of health-related outcomes
- The component parts of holistic measures are interrelated in that they interact to influence risk
- Holistic measures are powerful predictors of important health outcomes among youth, including self-rated health status and injury
- Young people's perceptions of their overall health status (a strong predictor of future morbidity and mortality) are determined by multiple domains of health, pointing to the importance of holistic approaches to health assessment and health promotion in this population

References

Adamson, P. (2010). *The children left behind: A league table of inequality in child well-being in the world's rich countries. Innocenti Report Card, no. 9.* Florence, Italy: UNICEF Innocenti Research Centre.

Bronfenbrenner, U. (1986). Ecology of the family as a context for human development: Research perspectives. *Developmental Psychology, 22*(6), 723–742.

Cantril, H. (1965). *The pattern of human concerns.* Rutgers, NJ: Rutgers University Press.

Christakis, N. A. (2012). Holism. In J. Brockman (Ed.), *This will make you smarter* (pp. 81–83). New York: Harper.

Currie, C., Gabhainn, S. N., Godeau, E., & International HBSC Network Coordinating Committee. (2009). The health behaviour in school-aged children: WHO collaborative cross-national (HBSC) study: Origins, concept, history and development 1982–2008. *International Journal of Public Health, 54*(2), 131–139.

DeSalvo, K. B., Bloser, N., Reynolds, K., He, J., & Muntner, P. (2006). Mortality prediction with a single general self-rated health question. *Journal of General Internal Medicine, 21*(3), 267–275.

Freeman, J., King, M., & Pickett, W. (2015). *Health behaviour in school-aged children (HBSC) in Canada: Focus on health relationships.* Ottawa, ON: Public Health Agency of Canada.

Hetland, J., Torsheim, T., & Aarø, L. E. (2002). Subjective health complaints in adolescence: Dimensional structure and variation across gender and age. *Scandinavian Journal of Public Health, 30*(3), 223–230.

Jessor, R. (1991). Risk behavior in adolescence: A psychosocial framework for understanding and action. *Journal of Adolescent Health, 12*(8), 597–605.

Joffer, J., Jerdén, L., Öhman, A., & Flacking, R. (2016). Explaining self-rated health among adolescents: A think-aloud study. *BMC Public Health, 16*(1), 156.

Kaplan, G. A., Goldberg, D. E., Everson, S. A., Cohen, R. D., Salonen, R., Tuomilehto, J., et al. (1996). Perceived health status and morbidity and mortality: Evidence from the Kuopio ischaemic heart disease risk factor study. *International Journal of Epidemiology, 25*(2), 259–265.

Kwong, J., Klinger, D.A., Janssen, I., Pickett, W. (2015). Adolescent risk-taking in Canada: A contemporary empirical study of the CDC framework. Queen's University, Kingston, ON: (Unpublished masters thesis).

Michaelson, V., Pickett, W., King, N., & Davison, C. (2016). Testing the theory of holism: A study of family systems and adolescent health. *Preventive Medicine Reports, 4,* 313–319.

Suhr, D. D. (2006). *Exploratory or confirmatory factor analysis?* (pp. 1–17). Cary: SAS Institute.

WHO. (1948). Preamble to the Constitution of the World Health Organization. In *Official Records of the World Health Organization, no. 2.* New York: International Health Conference.

Chapter 5
Integration of Findings

*Without integration, the knowledge yield is equivalent to that
from a qualitative study and a quantitative study undertaken
independently, rather than achieving a 'whole greater than the
sum of the parts'.*
—O'Cathain, Murphy & Nicholl

Abstract In this chapter, we use an intentional integration protocol in order to glean new understandings by considering both strands of enquiry (qualitative and quantitative) together. Emergent meta-themes from this process suggest that the theory of holism makes a valuable contribution to and has practical utility for the health of children. Further, balance is a high priority to the health of children, and holistic thinking is a useful way of facilitating balanced thinking. We also present interpretive insights about our thinking from key stakeholders, and discuss implications for health education, research and clinical care.

Keywords Holism · Mixed-methods · Triangulation · Integration

We began this short book by asking the question, "What makes a child healthy?" While all of the many facets of health—things like nutrition, social relationships, physical activity and emotional health—are important, we have argued that there is value, too, in considering child health in composite, or "as a whole". Throughout, we have applied multiple research approaches to explore this idea. When held together, what we have learned through both qualitative and quantitative strands of enquiry tells a compelling story about the potential utility of the theory of holism for contemporary thinking and practice around child health.

In this final chapter, we have two goals. The first is to integrate our qualitative and quantitative findings. This provides a fuller picture of what has been learned than could be gleaned from the use of one method in isolation. We do this by using a six-step integration protocol and applying it to a list of 16 agreed themes. Our second objective is to draw from all of our findings to suggest practical applications of the theory of holism to the broad fields of health education, health research and clinical care, as applied to children.

© The Author(s) 2018
V. Michaelson et al., *Holistic Health in Children: Conceptualization,
Assessment and Potential*, SpringerBriefs in Well-Being and Quality
of Life Research, DOI 10.1007/978-3-319-64831-6_5

Triangulation of Findings

Research that uses multiple methods to investigate the same research question has the advantage of maximizing the strengths of each method, while at the same time compensating for, or minimizing, respective weaknesses. This process of integration is called "triangulation".

The term triangulation originates from the sciences of land surveying and navigation, and refers to a simple method for determining the position of a point using observations from two additional points (Sharp, 1943). In mixed methods research, triangulation is often used to describe agreement between two or more sets of findings, but it can also be used to gain a more complete picture of a problem through the use of multiple methods (O'Cathain, Murphy, & Nicholl, 2010). The nature of the evidence generated by our studies render this second approach most applicable to our situation.

In this chapter, we follow a triangulation protocol developed by Farmer, Robinson, Elliott, and Eyles (2006). This approach permitted us, systematically, to integrate our findings so as to see if further insights could be gained by examining evidence from the qualitative and quantitative strands congruently. This standardized protocol has six steps, which we describe and discuss in turn below.

While this protocol was designed for use within studies involving multiple qualitative methods, we agree with O'Cathain et al. (p. 1148) that it is also relevant and useful to mixed methods projects. It involves developing a "convergence coding matrix", and displaying the findings from all strands on the same page. Researchers then consider where there is agreement, partial agreement, silence, or disagreement between findings from different components of the study. As researchers, this process enables us to move from thinking about the findings related to each method to identifying meta-themes that transcend the boundaries and the findings between methods. This systematic framework is valuable for comparing and contrasting our findings because it allows us, systematically, to see if further understanding about our topic of interest can be gained by looking at all the results together. Moreover, this integration helps us to look for meta-themes, and to understand the larger picture of our findings ourselves. Farmer et al., (2006) recommend that this process take place after both data sets have been analyzed separately, which was done in Chaps. 2, 3 and 4.

Six steps are included in this triangulation protocol.

Step 1—Sorting—Identifying key themes from both methodological strands
Step 2—Convergence Coding—Determining the level of agreement between two sets of results
Step 3—Convergence Assessment—Providing a global assessment of convergence of all segments
Step 4—Completeness Assessment—Comparing the scope of all unique topic areas

Step 5—Researcher comparison—Documenting where researchers had different opinions about convergence
Step 6—Feedback—Reviewing triangulated results with stakeholders.

Each step is described below.

Step 1—Sorting

Our first step was to identify key themes from both methodological strands, and to organize them into similar categories of findings. We reviewed evidence generated from the analyses described in Chaps. 2, 3 and 5, and identified the key emergent themes. We then created a unified list of findings, which formed the rows of a convergence-coding matrix (Farmer et al., 2006). In total, we identified 16 themes, which we then organized into five core categories:

1. Defining holism

   (i) Wholes have value that is different from and more than the sum of the parts
   (ii) The interconnections between the parts provide new insights into the whole
   (iii) Reductionism also has value
   (iv) Holistic thinking needs practical boundaries.

2. Child perceptions of health

   (v) Listening to the views of children is important
   (vi) Adult definitions of health can be perceived as inflexible by children
   (vii) Health is different for every person
   (viii) The customization of health has its limits.

3. Holistic metaphors

   (ix) Metaphors are useful tools for talking about health
   (x) Metaphors are flexible ways of talking about health
   (xi) Metaphors are useful for holistic thinking.

4. Holistic measurement

   (xii) It is possible to create holistic *measures* of health
   (xiii) Patterns and relationships become stronger when measured holistically
   (xiv) Patterns and relationships are more consistent when measured holistically
   (xv) It is possible to create holistic *models* of health.

5. Practical application

   (xvi) Methods for applying holistic thinking to child health can be applied in a large variety of contexts.

Step 2—Convergence Coding

Next, in order to integrate the findings of the two strands, we applied this coding scheme to explore similarities and differences between findings from the qualitative and quantitative strands. We categorized each meta-theme in terms of consistency of findings between the strands ("agreement"—*the two strands agree completely*, "partial agreement"—*the two strands agree in part*, "silence"—*no evidence on which to base any conclusions*, and "disagreement"—*evidence from the two strands disagreed*). Silence is expected, and is often explained by the strengths of the different methods to explore diverse aspects of a phenomenon. Disagreement, too, is anticipated, and may lead to a better understanding of the research question and further valuable insights (Bourgeault, Dingwall, & De Vries, 2010). This complete matrix is displayed below, in Table 5.1.

Each of the three researchers for this study filled out the matrix separately in order to determine convergence between the qualitative and quantitative results in relation to each theme. While the study used multiple methods both qualitatively and quantitatively, the matrix is organized not by study or analysis, but by the two broad methods as a whole.

When there was disagreement among the researchers, we had conversation and debate (see Step 5). One theme (theme 7), was identified as being both convergent and having disagreement.

Category 1: *Defining holism*: The first four themes in our convergence matrix are gathered under the category "defining holism", and relate to the core definition and

Table 5.1 Convergence matrix

Core theme	Agreement	Partial agreement	Silence	Disagreement
1. *Defining holism*				
(i) Wholes have value that is different from and more than the sum of the parts				
(ii). The interconnections between the parts provide new insights into the whole				
(iii). Reductionism also has value				
(vi) Holistic thinking needs practical boundaries				
2. *Child perceptions of health*				
v. Listening to the views of children is important, and yields unique insights				
vi. Adult definitions can be perceived as inflexible by children				
vii. Health is different for every person				
viii. The customization of health has its limits				
3. *Holistic metaphors*				
(ix) Metaphors are useful tools for talking about health				
(x) Metaphors are flexible ways of talking about health				
(xi) Metaphors are useful for holistic thinking				
4. *Holistic measurement*				
(xii) It is possible to create holistic *measurements* of health				
(xiii) Patterns and relationships become stronger when measured holistically				
(xiv) Patterns and relationships are more consistent when measured holistically				
(xv) It is possible to create holistic *models* of health				
5. *Practical application*				
xvi. Methods for applying holistic thinking can be applied in a variety of contexts				
Total	6	2	7	2

parameters of holism. We agreed fully that when it comes to the study of child health, both qualitative and quantitative methods demonstrated that wholes have value that is more than the sum of their component parts (theme 1). There was also agreement that the interconnections between the parts provide important new insights into the whole (theme 2). The third theme relates to reductionism—the idea that both component parts and their composites have value. This is perhaps best illustrated by our quantitative analysis of risk-taking and multiple risk behaviour. On their own, risk-taking behaviours appear to increase risk for injury and poor health in a consistent but not terribly compelling fashion. This is an important finding. But even more striking is the pattern observed when we examined these behaviours in a holistic way (through composite scores or even interactions). The trends are certainly still apparent, but they became much stronger. The recognition that a reductionist approach has value, but so too do the holistic findings, was reinforced through qualitative observations made by the young people themselves. The fourth theme relates to boundaries that need to be established in order to assess child health in a holistic yet practical manner. To illustrate, contextual influences are important in the shaping of one's health. These can include the effects of family, community and peer group dimensions. However, our attempts to incorporate these quantitatively into a summary measure were not terribly practical or informative. Instead, we had to focus on more proximal indicators of health in order to arrive at something measurable. Qualitatively, the natural boundaries offered by metaphors provided a practical framework for fruitful discussion.

Category 2: *Child perceptions of health*: The next four themes related to child perceptions of health. Theme 5 states that listening to the views of children is important, and yields unique insights. When analysing the convergence of findings on this theme between the qualitative and quantitative strands, there was initial disagreement between researchers as two researchers identified this as "silence" and the third researcher chose "partial agreement". On further discussion, one researcher made the argument that while qualitative inquiry directly asks children for their ideas, quantitative survey techniques do that as well, just in a more structured and less open-ended way. Even though the methods are different, both qualitative focus group data and quantitative questionnaire data entail listening to the voices of children. With conversation, we came to agreement on this viewpoint. We categorized this theme as "partial agreement" because we observed that the qualitative and quantitative findings offered complementary information on the same issue.

Theme 6 tells us that adult definitions can be perceived by children as inflexible. We categorized this as "silence", because while this was an important discussion point that emerged through our qualitative methods, it was not present in our quantitative study. This silence was not unexpected because this is an instance in which the two methods were being used for different purposes.

Theme 7 reports that health is different for everyone, and theme 8 conveys that "customized health has its limits". Theme 7 was an anomaly because we agreed that there was both agreement and disagreement between methods. Qualitatively, the children told us that health is "different for everyone". And yet, when we explored this idea in a quantitative manner, it was evident that children who were reporting

excellent health status were also reporting participation in a number of risk behaviours and other activities that are well established as being negative for health.
This is contradictory. Young people were very committed to the idea that one needs
to be flexible in determining the factors that constitute good health for an individual
person. However, there is a need for caution and perhaps healthy skepticism here,
which is central to our conversation around theme 8 that says that customized health
has its limits. Qualitatively, children did not perceive any limits to a customization
of health, and yet results from our quantitative strand suggested that while customized approaches to health can have value (for example, the self-rated health item
that we discussed in Chap. 4), such approaches need to be approached with caution.
Young people may have limited exposure to long-term consequences of unhealthy
decisions or the evidence base surrounding them, which may explain some of their
attitudes.

Category 3: *Holistic metaphors*: Themes 9, 10 and 11 each relate to metaphors.
All three researchers rated these three themes as "silence", which is somewhat easy
to explain. It is likely that the silence relates to differences in the focus, nature and
scope of the particular strands of the study, and also the strengths of both distinct
methodologies. We would not expect that quantitative methods would provide
insight into the use of metaphors, as that kind of exploration would be beyond the
scope of the method itself.

Category 4: *Holistic measurement*: Themes 13, 14 and 15 all relate to quantitative measurement, and again, having these themes identified by the researchers as
"silent" (or, unique to one strand of the study) is easily explained. It would not be
reasonable to expect qualitative methods to offer insight into quantitative patterns of
measurement used in this way. Note that we are not arguing that qualitative
methods do not have a place in measurement; only that statistical analysis of survey
questions and the kind of measuring instruments that were used in this study are not
used in parallel ways by qualitative researchers.

Theme 15 tells us that it is possible to create holistic models of health, and here
we chose "partial agreement". Our findings suggest that this is certainly true
quantitatively, as any model that involves scale development is somewhat holistic
in nature. When we asked children in our qualitative focus groups to approach
developing a model of health, at first they were a bit stumped. The real break-
through in thinking came when they proposed the use of metaphors. Once they
engaged with this concept, they capably and enthusiastically began to model their
own health using these methods. Therefore, while the investigators agreed that both
methods allow for holistic modeling of health, when this is done using qualitative
methods, there needs to be room both for flexibility and for the uniqueness of each
person to be expressed in the model.

Category 5: *Practical application*: Our final theme (16) relates to the practical
utility of applying the theory of holism to child health in a variety of contexts and
using a variety of methodological approaches. Here, too, we found agreement
between our qualitative and quantitative methods.

A summary model of this convergence coding is found here, in Fig. 5.1.

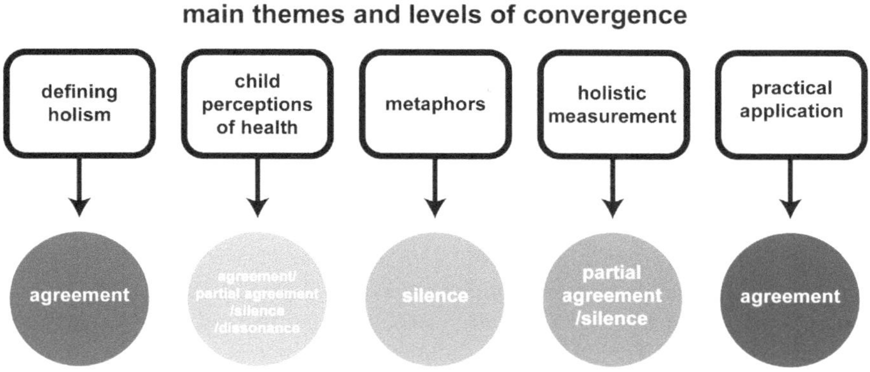

main themes and levels of convergence

Fig. 5.1 Summary model of main themes and level of convergence

Step 3—Convergence Assessment

Next we reviewed agreement within the entire matrix to determine a global assessment of the level of convergence. Our team of investigators concluded that there was full agreement between the qualitative and quantitative findings for 6/16 themes, partial agreement for 2/16, silence for 7/16, and dissagreement in 2/16. There was one theme (theme 7) for which both "agreement" and "dissagreement" were selected.

Step 4—Completeness Assessment

The purpose of the next step was to identify and focus on the unique themes that emerged through each study approach. There were eight instances in which we categorized themes as "silent" because only one of the methods highlighted these findings.

Given the nature and range of findings from both study approaches, silences in terms of agreement were not unexpected. Clearly, some research methods are better suited to addressing particular trends and experiences than others. Qualitatively, the focus groups deepened our understanding of how young people engage with health holistically. They demonstrated that using metaphors is a productive way of engaging with young people about holistic health. Our quantitative findings make a unique contribution by way of approaches to assessment and measurement, and enabled us to identify patterns and relationships, which we can then generalize to a large population group. The themes found in the category of silence identify the insights in our research question that would be missing had only one method-ological approach been used.

Step 5—Researcher Comparison

In Step 2 of the integration protocol, we did the convergence coding first as individuals and then as a team. There were two instances in which we had different perspectives on convergence or disagreement of findings (theme 5 and theme 15).

In both cases, we discussed the rationale behind the coding and added more detail and clarification in support of the themes. We came to consensus in both cases. The level of agreement between the researchers on the convergence coding of each of 16 themes was 87.5%. The level of agreement between researchers that is considered acceptable to ensure confidence in the coding process is 70% (Miles & Huberman, 1994), and our researcher agreement exceeded that. This gives us strong confidence in the convergence coding and completeness exercises.

Step 6—Feedback

The final step in our triangulation protocol was to seek feedback from community stakeholders. We identified community stakeholders, discussed findings and solicited feedback about the study as a whole and about our emergent meta-themes. Because of this, we report on their feedback after we have reported our meta-themes, in the section related to practical application below.

Summary of Integration and Identification of Meta-Themes

The six-step integration protocol enabled us to bring together multiple perspectives from complementary data sets related to our research question, and provided a more complete picture of the practical utility of holism to child health. The process helped us as researchers to move from thinking about the findings related to each method to identifying important meta-themes that transcend the boundaries and the findings of both methods. Figure 5.2 illustrates the three meta-themes that we identified through this integration process, and they are discussed below.

Fig. 5.2 Summary model of emergent meta-themes 1

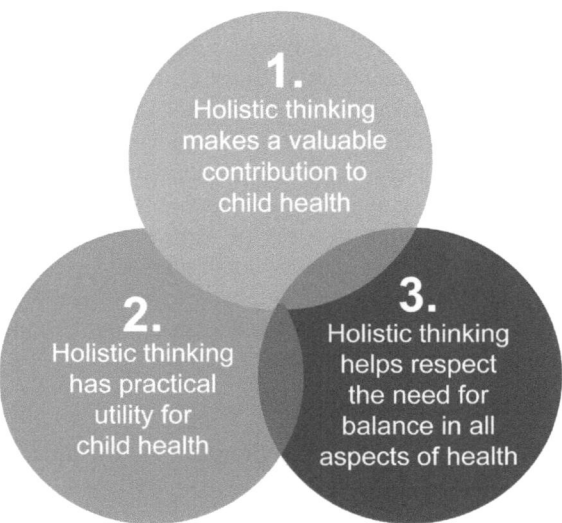

Meta-theme 1: Holistic Thinking Makes a Valuable Contribution to Child Health

When you look at children's health holistically, you see things that you would not see solely by looking at the parts (this includes a strengthening of patterns as well as the emergence of new ideas). Further, the interrelationship between the individual parts related to health becomes stronger or more apparent when health is looked at holistically, and this was confirmed regardless of which method we used. Whether health is being approached through the lens of education, research or clinical care, this kind of thinking yields important insights that might otherwise be missed.

Meta-theme 2: Holistic Thinking Has Practical Utility for Child Health

Not only does holistic thinking make a valuable contribution to child health, the theoretical concept of holism has practical utility for child health. It resonates strongly with young people, especially when it is used within a flexible framework such as metaphor. Metaphors in turn may offer a powerful pedagogical strategy for helping children to understand health holistically. Holism also has important applications to child health research.

Meta-theme 3: Holistic Thinking Helps Respect the Need for Balance in All Aspects of Health

Our third meta-theme is that holistic approaches are useful in facilitating approaches to children's health that respect the need for balance. Whether qualitative or quantitative methods are being used, when multiple aspects of health are looked at congruently, the risk of prioritizing one aspect of health over others is minimized. In part, this is because holistic approaches tend to highlight the importance of the many ways that the various parts work together. We are reminded again of the words of the 4th century (BCE) philosopher Socrates, which we presented in chapter one. He wrote, very simply, that "the part can never be well unless the whole is well" (Plato, 380 BCE). Whether we are talking about an individual child or a whole health system, a healthy balance between the parts is vital to the health of the whole. It is certainly useful for researchers, educators and practitioners to understand this concept. But inviting children to consider their own health in holistic ways is essential to understanding the consequences—both positive and negative—of health behaviours and choices. It also can offer children important insights about their own health that will help them to live well and fully in the context of their own lives.

Practical Applications for Holism and Child Health

Our ideas about holism are a small piece of a global conversation in which researchers, policy makers, educators and practitioners are exploring and articulating ways of thinking about health that look beyond the "bits and pieces" to the "whole". In this final section of our book, our goal is to apply what we have learned about the practical utility of holism for contemporary thinking and practice to health education, clinical care and health research.

During Step 6 of our integration protocol, we had the opportunity to talk with three professionals, who have hands-on applied experience related to various aspects of our study: Dr. Nancy Dalgarno, Education Researcher and Consultant, Office of Health Sciences Education/Department of Family Medicine-Centre for Studies in Primary Care, Queen's University; Dr. Susan Phillips, Clinical Practitioner, Queen's University Department of Family Medicine; and Mr. David Hannah, Educational Consultant, Bayridge Secondary School, Kingston, Canada. Their insights were extremely valuable to the practical application of our project, and we have included their voices in this section. Throughout this section, we also continue to recognize the voices of the many children who participated in our study.

Implications for Health Education

In Chap. 1, we reported that words like "holistic", "integrated", and "connected" are sprinkled throughout the Ontario Health Curriculum and represent important learning goals. But holism is an abstract concept, and it is not easy to teach. In Chaps. 2 and 3, we presented evidence as to why metaphors are useful ways of considering holistic health, and we suggested that metaphors may offer a fresh and creative pedagogical strategy for engaging children in considering their own health in holistic ways. But what do children think about this idea? We asked the same children who participated in the "Drawing Metaphors" study what they thought of this approach as a strategy for health education. Here is some of what they told us:

> I found that [working with the metaphors] was really interesting. It was an efficient and effective way to go about learning this. It is something that I can remember and it is really nice.

> Using metaphors was a good way [to get people our age thinking about health because] sometimes it is easier to understand things if you compare them to something else.

> It is easier to relate to metaphors because they are open to interpretation.

> If you give a solid definition it is like reading a dictionary and trying to connect to a dictionary.

> But if you were to use a metaphor you can interpret it in your own ways and connect with it in your own ways. So it is open to thought and you can kind of figure it out.

One participant told us about how he couldn't wait to tell his health teacher about the exercise, in hopes that he would continue building on the activity at school. He said

> Now that I have thought of this and I have brought this up, I think the next time I am talking about health in school, which will be probably next semester. So when we talk about health I will ask my teacher, 'Hey, how does this fit into my car engine idea?' And he will be like 'What is that?' And then I will explain it to him and hopefully I could help other students to maybe understand a bit better.

For our young participants, the metaphors were memorable. The child who worked with the Jenga metaphor even went so far as to tell us "I will keep the Jenga [metaphor] with me until the day I die". He was clearly being sarcastic when he said this, but it was equally clear that his Jenga metaphor had made a real impression on the way he now thought about his own health.

We asked the children in our study if it was important that we let them come up with their own metaphor or if it would have worked just as well if we had told them what to draw. The resounding response was that choosing their own metaphor was one of the most important parts of the exercise, because they could choose something that they personally connected with and also, "the more that your mind gets going makes it better". The child who had chosen the car engine explained why:

> The main reason I thought of the engine idea is because I have grown up around them throughout my life. My dad is a mechanic and the majority of his elders have been mechanics in their life. I have always been around them and I have always loved the idea of how things work and how they do the things they do. So the engine idea made the most sense. I have always loved it because each different part can't work without the other and is about your health in general. If you put two wheels with a rubber belt and take one of the wheels out, the rubber will just fall and spin around the one wheel. So it is not going to work as good as if it had another wheel to spin the rubber around and make sure that the health is going the way that it is supposed to or something like that. And if you take one of those things out then the health will not work as well as it should.

A second child then told us:

> In my case I don't do the sports or the cars. If you told us all to draw a car engine I would be like, how? And I wouldn't really understand what you were trying to get across because I don't do cars and they don't connect [with] me.

This third child explained the importance of choosing her own unique metaphor, and having the chance to develop it in her own way.

> I think if we had all started with this then we would have all had the same information and a lot of our drawings would have looked the same or similar. And then it wouldn't have really been our health. I think when we started by doing our own drawings then we all picked what was important for us and that is important for each person to do.

This strong preference for choosing their own metaphors as a basis for this activity fits with what others have found. For example, Talley (2011) writes that while metaphors can be generated by health workers, the media, or others, those that are most powerful are those originating from people's own lived experiences (Talley, p. 418). The children's enthusiasm in using metaphors to think about their own health, and the ways that metaphors are useful in helping children to understand the holistic and interconnected nature of health, suggest that metaphors could be very valuable for children's health education.

Mr. Hannah, one of the community stakeholders with whom we spoke, was not remotely surprised that the children responded to this activity in such a positive manner. He explained how in his own experiences in high schools, he has seen how children learn through metaphor by connecting old knowledge to new knowledge. This facilitates what he called "metacognition", a process by which students actually learn how to use their own brains to drive their own learning. In his mind, this kind of approach would be extremely useful to help children (from elementary school through high school) to connect the health curriculum with their own lived experiences. Both Dr. Dalgarno and Mr. Hannah agreed that while the idea of thinking about health holistically was reflective of the Ontario health curriculum, which both of them said was outstanding, what it really comes down to is the teacher in the classroom. Providing teachers with readily available and adaptable tools to teach health in holistic ways could be helpful.

Of course, any idea to make a curriculum around these teaching ideas would need to be tested, but our consultations with both of these stakeholders affirmed that this approach had a lot of potential. If this were tested and it were shown that indeed, this kind of approach does foster learning, it could be a very valuable tool to help children to understand the holistic and interconnected nature of their own health. Development of teacher tools that could then be tested would be a good starting place for such a project.

We reflected with both Dr. Dalgarno and Mr. Hannah about how a teacher could ask students to use a metaphor to draw their health at the beginning of the year (or semester), and with every unit, ask the children to continue to develop their pictorial metaphor of their own health. In this way, students would come to understand the way that every part of health relates to everything else. If one piece is missing there is a very good chance you will not be as healthy. Both of these experts agreed that this metaphor activity may also be a good way to address misconceptions the children have related to their own preconceptions, and to the ideas held by the young people that contradict the literature about adolescent health. As we discussed in Chaps. 2 and 3, young people's ideas about what is healthy for them do not always correlate with established evidence. If we do not also use opportunities such as health education in schools to introduce rigorous health research into children's ideas about health, there is a risk that children conceive health as anything they want it to be. Extremes are not helpful, and approaches that balance children's perspectives with rigorous research are optimal.

Implications for Health Research and Assessment

Our work also has implications for research and assessment. Using quantitative methods, we found that if we don't look at the whole, we might miss something important. The strength and consistency of emergent relationships are not evident in reductionist models, which suggests that there is some truth in this perspective. Rarely are health-related exposures found in isolation; rather they exist as part of a larger holistic system with interacting parts. This is particularly true in the social sciences, but is true of other disciplines as well.

The final stakeholder with whom we consulted was Dr. Phillips, who is both a health researcher and a family doctor. She reflected on our findings with some cautionary words. Her perspective was that if, as a doctor, she takes up all the time on the big picture, she could quite easily miss a diagnosis. Too much time looking at the whole might well mean missing an important component that contributes to health and disease. In medicine, knowing the whole child but missing the diagnosis is an unacceptable approach. But at the same time, she also told us that one needs to know the child in order to make the diagnosis and figure out appropriate treatment, which comes back to the one-on-one relationship between doctor and patient. Her reflections as a family medicine practitioner were very thoughtful:

> Medically, when I see a child I can't help but think about the whole person. I always think of the person in context. If I didn't do that, would I be worse at diagnosing something like strep throat? Probably not. It wouldn't change my diagnoses. I don't know how to bring holistic thinking into diagnostics, but it is essential to talking to patients. That is where holistic approaches show the most.

Her words reminded us of Freeman's work on holistic health in which he explains that an implicit part of the comprehensive care provided by general practitioners is necessarily holistic. He writes:

> We are not doctors for particular diseases, or particular organs, or particular states in the life cycle – we are doctors for people. People are complex, and live in complex communities in a complex world. All aspects of this world have an impact on the health of the people in it (2005, p. 155).

This is perhaps why the European Academy of Teachers of General Practice (EURACT, 2002), identified holistic modeling' as one of the 'six core competencies of the GP/family doctor' (Freeman, 2005).

Clearly, there needs to be a balance between holistic and reductionist approaches. The potential pitfall of reductionist approaches in quantitative research is that this 'system' can be ignored, or not appropriately modeled. As a result, we may not be fully explaining the nature of the relationship between the exposure and outcome. In such instances, more holistic approaches may be necessary.

We began this study with the realization that today's children may conceptualize health in ways that do not fit into historical paradigms. Because of this, qualitative methods that listen to children's views and perspectives are essential in helping us to understand, from a child's perspective, the importance of the things we are measuring. Qualitative work can also inform what might go into a holistic measure in various contexts, and reminds us of the flexibility required to reflect the different needs of different children. Dr. Phillips echoed the importance of listening to children intentionally so that we truly understand their perspectives and concerns. As a practitioner, she talked about how easy it is to let parents talk for their kids. But, as she listened to children in her own practice, she realized how rich an interaction is possible if children are given a voice. For her, the idea that children have their own ideas and insights and need to be listened to is a very important message for medicine.

We had approached our study on holistic measurement with the view that it would be useful for epidemiological health research, but educator David Hannah suggested that they might also have application to student assessment. In our interview, he speculated as to whether holistic thinking, and these ideas about measurement, could help to develop a scale that aligns with what public education should do. In his mind, this is to equally value academic achievement with resilience, perseverance, collaboration and kindness (or the two sides of the report card). "It's hard to put a quantitative value on human dignity", he said, "which is unfortunate". He told us very simply that the "kids care about what the adults care about," and "when they see that the marks we value most are for academic success, that becomes the priority for them as well. So rather than try to flourish as whole human beings, the children try to get good marks."

Mr. Hannah was reflective. In the decades that he has worked as a high school teacher in Ontario, he told us he has been uncomfortable with assessment. In looking at our work in holistic measurement, he mused out loud: "Could we rethink assessment in school to better reflect the whole child?" For Mr. Hannah, a disconnect comes with all of the curricular pressures; it is too easy to focus on doing well at school rather than doing well as human beings. For him, and we expect for most teachers, those two things—academic success and thriving as a whole human being—should not be at odds. But because the world we live in is so quick, and we are always so distracted, it is too easy to fall into the trap of separating those goals. Though abstract, holism is also extremely simple. To Mr. Hannah, that's why these ideas are so vital for today's kids. "Our problems are complex," he said "but it doesn't mean our solutions have to be."

Wider Implications

In Chap. 1, we reviewed ways that holistic thinking is already recognized as important in many policy contexts. From many Indigenous health policies (AFN, 2013) to policy frameworks such as the Mandala of Health and the Wider Determinants of Health Model, it is not uncommon for policies to recognize the multiple and diverse factors that simultaneously influence health. The holistic approaches to quantitative measurement that we have presented could be valuable ways to measure and monitor the effectiveness of these policy frameworks.

The qualitative model of using metaphors to engage with children about health in holistic ways potentially offers a means of communicating health policies or health promotion initiatives in ways that resonate with children. Talley already points to how the power of metaphor "is reflected in their emerging place as formal tools in the public health toolbox." (pg 416 Talley), and so it is perhaps no surprise that it could be a powerful tool for communicating with children. However, before metaphors were adopted as a vehicle for communicating various health information to young people, this idea would need to be formally tested.

We were attentive to two words of caution that were offered by Dr. Phillips. First, she raised concerns that medicine has accepted the body as machine metaphor, thinking that the parts define the whole and that failing parts can be repaired, removed or replaced without changing 'the whole'. And second, she pointed out that while the concept of holism is powerful and important, the word has become tainted by alternative messages and should be used with caution. One way to address this problem would be to choose another word that has been less tainted, but it is not obvious what that word would be. A second strategy would be to do as we have already proposed, and that is to carefully define and draw boundaries around the word holism and holistic in relation to health so that it can be used well. We hope that in this book, this is what we have done.

Drs. Dalgarno and Phillips both noted that the priority of balance was perhaps the most important of our findings. For Dr. Phillips, balance is about not maximizing nor minimizing a patient's problems, but keeping a balanced approach. She talked about finding a balance between "content" (what's inside you) and "context" (the world in which you live), and how both are important to clinical care. And for Dr. Dalgarno, in the fast-paced and fully programed world in which today's adolescents live and interact, "many children need balance more than just about anything." Further, she advised us that perhaps our study was much more interconnected than our initial model (Fig. 5.2) demonstrated. She speculated that there was greater overlap between our themes, and on reflection, we adjusted our final model of meta-themes to reflect this balance more fully (Fig. 5.3).

Fig. 5.3 Summary model of emergent meta-themes 2

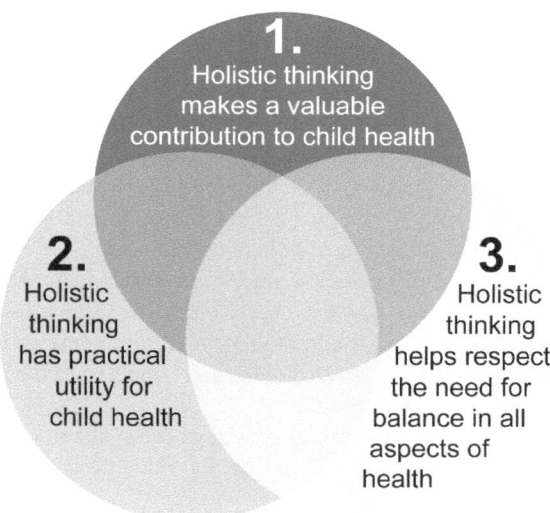

1.
Holistic thinking makes a valuable contribution to child health

2.
Holistic thinking has practical utility for child health

3.
Holistic thinking helps respect the need for balance in all aspects of health

Strengths and Challenges of this Integration Protocol

Strengths and challenges of this integration protocol warrant comment. One strength is that using an intentional triangulation strategy adds to the validity of interpretations, and enables researchers to bring together multiple perspectives on a particular research question. This systematic process enabled us to probe different elements of our research question, and provide complementary findings that in turn, led to a more complete understanding of our research question.

The data from the quantitative and qualitative strands of this study serve different purposes and as a result, the shape of their content is different. While this is a strength, it is also a limitation because it is difficult to determine agreement on findings. For example, if a theme is absent in one data set and present in another, or if there is disagreement on findings between data sets, it is challenging to determine if these differences are due to the nature of the research method, the focus of the data collection, or legitimate differences in findings (Farmer et al., 2006). A second challenge relates to interpreting the importance of findings from different strands of the study. Because some forms of data may be more aptly suited to addressing a particular research question, findings from one set of data may be privileged over the other during triangulation. A final challenge during triangulation is to ensure that the findings from each set are presented at a similar level of detail, which we have tried to do throughout this book (Farmer et al., 2006).

Conclusion

Holism is a theoretical framework for talking about health that is increasingly being recognized as important for improving our health. Rarely has this concept been considered specifically with children in mind. Our overall goal in this book was to consider the potential of the theoretical concept of holism to support child health in practical ways. In Chaps. 2 and 3, we confirmed that the idea of holistic health resonates with young people, and that it is a useful way to help young people to think about health in the contemporary world. We also developed a useful and effective way of engaging young people in applying holistic thinking to their own health through the use of metaphors. In Chap. 4, we provided further evidence to an emergent, contemporary conversation that it is possible to assess health holistically in a quantitative manner, and offered four examples of how this can be done. We demonstrated that when holistic measurement tools are used, the strength and consistency of relationships is even stronger, and the relationships between the parts are more fully understood.

Overall, we offer further evidence for the practical value of holism for child health. Certainly, it will always be valuable to study individual components that contribute to health. But when health is looked at holistically, we see things that we would not see otherwise—be that strength of relationships or new ideas altogether. Examining health holistically also provides new insights into the way that the parts interact and depend on each other. Finally, holism provides insight into balance: balance between various approaches to health (adult voices and child voices) and also balance between various aspects of health (for example, physical and social health). Beyond being a vague word in various curricula and policies, holism is a concept that could concretely inform health research and education, and may also have important application for health policy and health promotion

In Chap. 1, we saw that the etymology of the word *health* itself offers a clue that health is inherently holistic. There is a sense that health is about being whole, not only in our bodies, but in our minds, in our spirits, in our relationships, and beyond. Throughout this book, we have seen a variety of constructs of health, and notably many of them have been Indigenous, that remind us that health is about more than bodies and disease. Holistic thinking pushes the ways that many people think about health to include generosity, human dignity, community and belonging. Indeed, in some contexts, health could even be considered the journey of becoming whole human beings.

Plato wrote that health is more than a healthy body. It is an integration of body and soul; "it is a vision of the good life itself" (Stempsey, 2001, p. 209). Other holistic views of health offer similar insights. Indigenous views of health remind us of the importance of regaining balance in our lives. And additional understandings of health such as Shalom and Ubuntu recognize that health is about being whole, not only in our bodies but as whole human beings, and remind us that we are most healthy when we are flourishing in the matrix of relationships that shape our lives. As we wrote in Chap. 1, these sorts of holistic approaches push our ideas about health beyond scientifically measureable constructs (such as height, weight, social capital and relative affluence) to attributes of kindness, vulnerability and belonging.

In Chap. 1, we shared the image of a birthday cake as a metaphor for holism. Christakis (2012) points to another example of holism that is even more impressive: life. He writes:

> carbon, hydrogen, oxygen, nitrogen, sulfur, phosphorus, iron, and a few other elements, when mixed in just the right way, yield life. And life has emergent properties not present in —nor predictable from—these constituent parts. There is a kind of awesome synergy between the parts (p. 81).

Grappling with the relationship between the properties of the individual parts, Christakis observes that the properties of the atoms—such as darkness and softness, clarity and hardness, are not properties of carbon atoms themselves, but are properties of the collection of atoms, and moreover, depend entirely on how they are assembled. For Christakis, this is a stunning example of holism, and "crucial" for a proper scientific perspective on the world. But he takes us further still. "You could know everything about isolated neurons and not be able to say how memory works, or where desire originates" (p. 82). Here again, the whole is more than the sum of the parts, and the whole creates something that cannot be entirely explained, no matter how much effort goes into reducing it and analyzing the individual parts.

This integrative approach reflects holism at its core, and harkens back to the rich and holistic heritage of health. Here in the 21st century, both Einstein's and Smuts' instincts that holism would have an important contribution to human thinking have certainly begun to be realized. With this in mind, we reiterate that while individual components of child health are valuable to understand, we need to put the child back together again. The emergent picture provided by a more holistic approach may be bigger than the sum of its parts, and is important to understand.

The fundamental goal of our efforts to view child health in a holistic manner is to understand what children need in order to live well and fully in the context of their everyday lives. Use of such thinking provides opportunities for new insights into health and its determinants in adolescents.

We began this book by asking the question, "What makes a child healthy?" While all of the many components—things like nutrition, social relationships, physical activity and emotional health—are important, what we have argued is that there is value, too, in considering child health in an integrative and whole fashion. Throughout this small book, we have applied multiple research approaches to explore this idea. When held together, what we have learned through both qualitative and quantitative methods tells a compelling story about the practical utility of holism for contemporary thinking and practice around child health.

Key Insights from This Chapter

- Qualitative and quantitative research methods both provide insights into using holism to think about child health
- When the emergent findings from both methods are integrated, we are given a more complete perspective on our research question

Key Findings

- We used a triangulation protocol to facilitate this integration. Meta-themes included:
  - Holism makes a valuable contribution to child health
  - Holism has practical utility for child health
  - Balance is a high priority in child health and holism is a useful way of thinking that facilitates balance

Practical Application

- The ideas presented in this book have practical application to many aspects of child health including health education, clinical care and health research

References

AFN. (2013). *First Nations holistic policy and planning a transitional discussion document on the social determinants of health.* Ottawa, Ontario: Assembly of First Nations. Retrieved from http://health.afn.ca/uploads/les/sdoh_afn.pdf.

Bourgeault, I., Dingwall, R., & De Vries, R. (Eds.). (2010). *The SAGE handbook of qualitative methods in health research.* London, UK: Sage. http://health.afn.ca/uploads/les/sdoh_afn.pdf.

Christakis, N. A. (2012). Holism. In J. Brockman (Ed.), *This will make you smarter* (pp. 81–83). New York: Harper.

EURACT. (2002). *The EURACT educational agenda of general practice/family medicine.* Retrieved from http://www.bibliosgam.ch/pdf/euract_agenda.pdf.

Farmer, T., Robinson, K., Elliott, S. J., & Eyles, J. (2006). Developing and implementing a triangulation protocol for qualitative health research. *Qualitative Health Research, 16*(3), 377–394.

Freeman, J. (2005). Towards a definition of holism. *The British Journal of General Practice, 55* (511), 154–155.

Miles, M. B., & Huberman, A. M. (1994). *Qualitative data analysis* (2nd ed.). Thousand Oaks, CA: Sage.

O'Cathain, A., Murphy, E., & Nicholl, J. (2010). Three techniques for integrating data in mixed methods studies. *BMJ, 341,* c4587. doi:10.1136/bmj.c4587.

Plato. (380 BCE). *Charmides.* Retrieved from http://classics.mit.edu/Plato/charmides.html.

Sharp, H. O. (1943). *Photogrammetry* (3rd ed.). New York, NY: John.

Stempsey, W. E. (2001). Plato and holistic medicine. *Medicine, Health Care and Philosophy, 4*(2), 201–209.

Talley, J. (2011). Metaphor, narrative, and the promotion of public health. *Genre, 44*(3), 405–423.

Appendix A
Full Methods for "Child Perceptions of Health" Qualitative Study (Chapter 2)

Grounded Theory Approach

The first qualitative study, Child Perceptions of Health (reported in Chap. 2), followed the qualitative, constant comparative method of grounded theory (Glaser & Strauss, 1967). This method requires the project to begin with an area of interest rather than a preconceived theoretical perspective. By adhering to this principle, the particular research problem and the theory used to account for the social phenomena are conceived "from the ground up" (Charmaz, 2014, p. 125). We began with a general interest in youth perceptions of health, and wondered how young people would resonate with ideas about holistic health (or as we described it in the study, "the health of a whole person"). Data were generated as we asked open-ended questions related to this topic in focus groups of young people aged 11–15 years. During this process, the investigators were simultaneously involved in both data collection and analysis, and hence mid-collection analysis shaped following data collection procedures. As theories began to emerge throughout initial coding and analyses, subsequent questions were then modified and became more focused. Data collected in the early stages of the study permitted us to compile more evidence around emerging themes and questions. In the early data collection efforts of this broader study, a significant theme emerged regarding using metaphors as a vehicle for talking about health with children. As interviewers, we focused questions iteratively in order to explore this theme more fully throughout subsequent data collection. The use of the iterative strategies of constant comparison and memoing ensured that the emergent theory was grounded in the data.

Recruitment and Participants

Participants were recruited using a purposeful, criterion-based approach. Participants who shared one or more criteria (including age, sex, rural/urban geographic status and immigration status) were recruited. Homogenous groups of like participants (i.e. all boys, all girls, etc.) were formed in order to facilitate conversation, and diversity was achieved between groups. Our final sample included seven

© The Author(s) 2018

V. Michaelson et al., *Holistic Health in Children: Conceptualization,
Assessment and Potential*, SpringerBriefs in Well-Being and Quality
of Life Research, DOI 10.1007/978-3-319-64831-6

focus groups, whose members were selected from populations in Eastern Ontario (Hastings and Frontenac Counties), Northern Ontario (Greater Sudbury), Western Ontario (Bruce County) and the Greater Toronto Area. A total of 40 young people were involved. All participants were recruited using "snowball" or "chain" sampling (Patton, 2001). Letters of information and informed consent were given to well-situated people who we predicted might be aware of potential participants, with the request to circulate the study information in their community. Recruitment was considered complete when the core question was saturated. Saturation does not imply that novel ideas would not emerge with additional data collection; rather, it suggests that sufficiently rich and dense data have been collected to enable an adequate understanding of key concepts (Charmaz, 2014).

Data Collection

Data collection was conducted within the seven focus groups. Focus group methods were an especially appropriate methodology for this study in that they are highly flexible and practical, they permit the gathering of large amounts of information in relatively short periods of time, and they may reveal concepts that previously have not been considered by the researcher (Babbie, 2007). Furthermore, focus groups enable researchers to better understand how members of a group arrive at, or alter their opinions or conclusions about, some topic or issue as they communicate. Focus groups do not require complex sampling strategies, and the facilitator can explore related but unanticipated topics as they emerge (Patton, 2001). Potentially sensitive topics may appear to be less threatening to participants when activities and tasks are incorporated into the focus group sessions (Berg, 2009).

Participants were given the opportunity to interact with standard definitions of health that were selected because although they reflect different ways of approaching health, they each incorporate ideas that could be considered holistic. We wondered if the participants would resonate with any of the definitions, or if they would find them useful tools for talking about health. The definitions were:

1. Health is "the capacity of people to adapt to, respond to, or control life's challenges and changes" (Frankish, Green, Ratner, Chomik, & Larsen, 1996).
2. "Health is a state of complete physical, mental and social well-being and not merely the absence of disease or infirmity" (World Health Organization, 1948).
3. "Health is a resource for daily living"(Government of Canada, 2014).

Children were asked, "Are there any words you would like to add or take away?" and "Do any of these definitions resonate with you more than the others?" Open ended-questions were used in order to invite rich discussion from each group. One sample question asked was this: "When you think of a healthy person, what are the first words that comes to your mind?"

Modelling health Step 1
"What Does Health Look Like in a Whole Person?"

After this initial discussion about definitions, we asked participants to imagine what health would look like "in a whole person". To fuel discussion, we used photo elicitation techniques (Harper, 2002). This is a research technique in which visual images are used to elicit ideas and discussion. The key element in photo elicitation is "not the form of the visual representation, but its relationship with the culture under study" (Harper, 2002, p. 19). Sixty images were selected by the researchers and presented to a pilot group of children prior to the study. Each card reflected one or more of what we thought might be interpreted as a wide range of aspects of health, including physical, emotional, social and spiritual health. Photographs that might elicit conversation about the contexts that young people are exposed to and could influence and determine health were also chosen. These included images depicting aspects of poverty, affluence, school environments, home environments, and neighbourhoods, and images showing the larger environmental context of our planet. The 40 images that generated the most meaningful conversation during the pilot group were then selected for the study.

Although photographs do not automatically elicit useful conversation, when used effectively, they have the power to capture an element of human consciousness or experience that is different from and complementary to "words-alone" interviews. This has been attributed to the way that remembering is enhanced by visual prompts (Harper, 2002). Because using predetermined photos introduced an element of preformed ideas about health into our study, this study is described as "grounded theory inspired" in that it lacks the complete openness of grounded theory. Regardless, even when using predetermined images, participants will see the images subjectively and bring their own experiences and ideas into the conversation (Flick, Von Kardorff, & Steinke, 2004). Photo elicitation is a powerful tool in that it may further facilitate meaningful conversation by anchoring the conversation in an image that is understood, at least in part, by all parties and is external to any one individual. This allows new interpretation and different perspectives to emerge.

From the full set of 40 picture cards, we gave each participant a deck of 5–8 cards. A sample question used for this activity was "How does one of the cards that you have help you to describe an aspect of being healthy or unhealthy?" The children were asked to choose a picture that helped them to talk about their ideas, or to share something different that was not reflected by a card. The interviewers provided an opportunity for participants to reject any of the cards if they did not feel that they related to health. There was also an opportunity for new and unanticipated themes to emerge from the discourse, and participants were asked to think about any further aspects of health that were not reflected by the cards.

Modelling Health Step 2
Organizing the Aspects of Health into Categories

The next step in our study was to ask participants to organize the various aspects of health into different categories that would reflect the health of a whole person, and to give each category a descriptive name. Each group approached this task slightly differently, though there was overlap in many of the categories that they identified.

Modelling Health Step 3
Organizing the Categories into the Health of a Whole Person

After the categories were established, we transcribed the names of each category onto 8-inch translucent circles. We then invited participants to organize the circles into a model that would "show us what health looks like all together in a whole person their age".

Coding and Analysis

A verbatim transcript of all focus group interviews was created by a professional transcriber. Data were coded (or organized into key conceptual themes) primarily by two researchers. At first working independently, these two researchers reviewed several transcripts in order to determine preliminary coding structures for organizing the data thematically. Initially, open and descriptive codes were applied. A second level of axial coding was then applied, which resulted in the identification of higher level, more conceptual categories. This multistage approach to coding helped to provide an in-depth understanding of how young people conceptualize health in holistic ways.

Academic Rigor

Throughout analysis, we employed tools of constant comparison, theoretical sensitivity and triangulation. These techniques ensured that all codes, categories and themes were grounded in the data. Constant comparison helped to ensure that each piece of data was considered in relation to previous and subsequent data, and that data was not fragmented but considered as a whole. Throughout the coding and analysis process, we also used theoretical memoing in order to record additional insights, questions and themes. Furthermore, as ideas emerged, they were compared with previous and subsequent interviews. The interview guide was modified iteratively based on the analysis of previous interviews, which was done in order to probe more deeply into the codes and theories that emerged. Multiple researchers engaged in critical dialogue around all aspects of data collection, coding and analysis, which further enhanced the rigour of the study and minimized individual researcher bias.

Ethical Considerations

This study received ethics approval from the Queen's University Health Sciences & Affiliated Teaching Hospitals Research Ethics Board (approval number EPID-447-13 ROMEO/TRAQ #6011166). All parents provided written, informed consent and all participants gave written and verbal informed assent prior to participation in the study.

Strengths and Limitations

This study has many strengths. Along with providing further understanding about how holistic health is perceived by children, we provided the opportunity for young people to have a voice in our program of research. Participants in the focus groups were articulate and engaged. The resultant data are textured, deep and nuanced, and observations were honestly and generously shared. Because our study focused on questions that had significant practical value, the thoughts and ideas that participants shared were rooted in their real-life experiences. Participants came from a variety of age groups, and represented the views of both genders and a diversity of school, socio-economic and family experiences. Though two-thirds of the focus group participants were girls, the themes that emerged in our focus group that was exclusively boys were consistent with results from the full sample. This study gives voice to a sample of young people and in this way, makes a significant contribution to conversations around children's health. Qualitative findings provided rich contextual understanding of youth perceptions of health, and enabled us to include a genuine youth voice.

While we are excited about the findings from this study, it is not without limitations. First, it is limited geographically to the province of Ontario, Canada, and hence may not be generalizable across populations and places. Because focus groups may be dominated by one or two personalities, some children may not have felt comfortable sharing their own opinions honestly. This danger was, however, mitigated somewhat by the experienced facilitators who were trained to build rapport and enable each person's voice to be heard. Finally, all participants were first approached about participation through their parent(s). This may have led to a positive bias in that children with a positive parent/child relationship may have been more likely to agree to participation and children with poor parent/child relationships may not have been approached or may have declined participation.

References

Babbie, E. (2007). *The practice of social research* (11th ed.). Belmont, CA: Wadsworth.
Berg, B. L., & Lune, H. (2009). *Qualitative research methods for the social sciences* (7th ed.). Boston, MA: Allyn & Bacon.
Charmaz, K. (2014). *Constructing grounded theory*. London, UK: Sage.
Flick, U., Von Kardorff, E., & Steinke, I. (2004). *A companion to qualitative research*. London, UK: Sage.
Frankish, C. J., Green, L. W., Ratner, P. A., Chomik, T., & Larsen, C. (1996). *Health impact assessment as a tool for population health promotion and public policy: A report submitted to the health promotion division of Health Canada. Institute of Health Promotion Research.* Vancouver, BC: University of British Columbia.
Glaser, B. G., & Strauss, A. L. (1967). *The discovery of grounded theory*. Chicago, IL: Aldine.
Government of Canada. (2014). *Health behaviour in school-aged children in Canada: Focus on relationships. Public Health Agency of Canada.* Retrieved from http://healthycanadians.gc.ca/publications/science-research-sciences-recherches/health-behaviour-children-canada-2015-comportements-sante-jeunes/index-eng.php#x.
Harper, D. (2002). Talking about pictures: A case for photo elicitation. *Visual Studies, 17*(1), 13–26. doi: 10.1080/14725860220137345.
Patton, M. Q. (2001). *Qualitative research and evaluation methods* (3rd ed.). London, UK: Sage.
World Health Organization. (1948). *WHO definition of health*, preamble to the constitution of the World Health Organization as adopted by the International Health Conference, New York, 19–22 June 1946; signed on 22 July 1946 by the representatives of 61 States (official records of the World Health Organization, no. 2, p. 100) and entered into force on 7 April 1948. In Grad, Frank P. (2002). "The Preamble of the Constitution of the World Health Organization." *Bulletin of the World Health Organization. 80*(12): 982.

Appendix B
Full Methods for "Children's Drawings of Metaphors" Qualitative Study (Chapter 3)

Here we report full methods for the qualitative study reported in Chap. 3, "Using children's drawing of metaphors to explore holistic health". Because it was complementary, and built on the first study that we reported in Chap. 2, we used many similar methodological strategies.

Overview of Approach

This second study used arts-based drawing techniques to elicit conversation and to compile new evidence. Based on other studies that have used drawing techniques (Onyango-Ouma, Aagaard-Hansen, & Jensen, 2004; Pridmore & Bendelow, 1995; Piko & Back; Psych, & Larsen, 2004), we expected that the use of illustrative drawings would enable children to express their ideas at their own levels, and provide a helpful springboard for engaging with ideas about holistic health. This method is child-centred, and demonstrates a respect for children and the importance of listening to their views (DiCarlo, Gibbons, Kaminsky, Wright, & Stiles, 2000; Merriman & Guerin, 2006).

Data Collection

Recruitment and Participants

Participants were recruited using a purposeful approach. All participants were boys and girls between 11 and 15 years old who lived in Eastern Ontario. A total of 19 children were involved (7 boys and 11 girls). All participants were recruited using "snowball" or "chain" sampling (Patton, 2001). Letters of information and informed consent were given to well-situated people who we predicted might be aware of

© The Author(s) 2018
V. Michaelson et al., *Holistic Health in Children: Conceptualization, Assessment and Potential*, SpringerBriefs in Well-Being and Quality of Life Research, DOI 10.1007/978-3-319-64831-6

potential participants, with the request to circulate the study information in their community.

Introducing Metaphors

We began by introducing examples of metaphors to the children ("those sisters are two peas in a pod" or "your room is a disaster area!"), and found that all participants had at least some familiarity with such expressions.

Drawing Health Step 1
"Draw Your Health"

After introducing the concept of metaphors, we provided paper and a variety of sizes and colours of felt markers, and asked participants to use one of those metaphors (or another metaphor, if they preferred) to "draw your health". We did not give directions around what we meant by "your health", and if asked we simply said "however you understand your health, that's what you draw". We told them that they would have multiple chances to discuss, add to and even change their drawings all together if they so chose. The children drew for about 15 minutes, and we then asked them to share and discuss what they had drawn.

Drawing Health Step 2
Presenting Infographics and Fact Sheets

Our next step was to present the children with "infographics" and "fact sheets" that summarized evidence about health and its determinants, including information around nutrition, sleep, physical activity, bullying, healthy relationships and mental health. Our purpose was to invite the children to consider their own drawings in light of this new information. The children could then decide if they wanted to develop or modify their drawings based on the new information.

We introduced this exercise by stating "Here are some things that adults (including doctors and researchers) tell us are important to good health in people your age". We asked them to consider if anything they had learned belonged in their picture, and if so, to incorporate it into their drawing. We gave them 15 minutes to think and draw, and then asked them to report on whether and how their picture (or metaphor) had evolved.

Drawing Health Step 3
Presenting Whole Pictures of Health

Finally, we encouraged the children to think about their metaphor as a whole picture of health rather than solely to focus on the individual parts. We also gave each child a set of pictures to consider. Instead of more infographics, these pictures now reflected existing holistic models of health. They included the Indigenous medicine wheel, an ecological model of health designed for children, and a picture of the earth. We then asked the participants to consider whether or not these pictures helped them to think of something they wanted to add to their drawing or helped them to see their drawings differently.

Coding and Analysis

A verbatim transcript of both focus groups was created by a professional transcriber. Line-by-line coding of the transcript then enabled us to identify each participant's ideas that emerged throughout the focus group. We use the children's pictures illustratively throughout Chap. 3. However, the actual interpretation of the pictures was done through analysis of the focus group transcripts of the children's interpretations of their own pictures, and not through our study of the pictures themselves. This approach is respectful of the young people and their ideas, and protects the investigators from misinterpreting the children's visual ideas.

We analyzed audio transcripts of the study by each individual study step (step 1, step 2, step 3). Within that framework, we used line-by-line coding to identify important themes emergent in the discussion for each step.

Ethical Considerations

This study received ethics approval from the Queen's University Health Sciences & Affiliated Teaching Hospitals Research Ethics Board (approval number EPID-447-13 ROMEO/TRAQ #6011166). All parents provided written, informed consent and all participants gave written and verbal informed assent prior to participation in the study.

Strengths and Limitations

Strengths of this study include the use of drawing pictures as a powerful way of understanding children's experiences. Our study allowed children to root their ideas about health into their own, lived-experiences, and because of this, our study had real practical value. Although participants came from one community in Ontario, they reflect a variety of age groups, and represent the views of both genders and a diversity of school, socio-economic and family experiences.

One challenge and potential limitation in analysis related to how we would interpret the children's drawings, which is difficult to do in a reliable manner (Thomas & Jolley, 1998). To mitigate this, we used our transcript of the audio recording of each focus group as the primary basis for interpretation of the children's work. Here, children described their own drawings in detail, reflected on the different choices they had made, and often commented on the work of their peers. As much as possible, we reported their ideas verbatim. Because we used the children's own descriptions of their pictures as our mode of analysis, we are confident that we have described the pictures in the ways that the children intended.

Other limitations of our study are similar to those we reported in Appendix A, for our first qualitative investigation. First, this study was limited geographically to a community in Eastern Ontario, Canada, and hence may not be generalizable across populations and places. Because focus groups may be dominated by one or two personalities, some children may not have felt comfortable sharing their own opinions honestly. This danger was, however, mitigated somewhat by the experienced facilitators who were trained to build rapport and enable each person's voice to be heard. Finally, all participants were first approached about participation through their parents. Again, this may have led to a positive bias in that children with a positive parent/child relationship may have been more likely to agree to participation and children with poor parent/child relationships may not have been approached or may have declined participation.

References

DiCarlo, M. A., Gibbons, J. L., Kaminsky, D. C., Wright, J. D., & Stiles, D. A. (2000). Street children's drawings: Windows into their life circumstances and aspirations. *International Social Work, 43,* 107–120.

Merriman, B., & Guerin, S. (2006). Using children's drawings as data in child-centred research. *The Irish Journal of Psychology, 27*(1–2), 48–57.

Onyango-Ouma, W., Aagaard-Hansen, J., & Jensen, B. B. (2004). Changing concepts of health and illness among children of primary school age in Western Kenya. *Health Education Research, 19*(3), 326–339.

Piko, B. F., & Bak, J. (2006). Children's perceptions of health and illness: Images and lay concepts in preadolescence. *Health Education Research, 21*(5), 643–653.

Pridmore, P., & Bendelow, G. (1995). Images of health: Exploring beliefs of children using the 'draw-and-write' technique. *Health Education Journal, 54*(4), 473–488.

Psych, C., & Larsen, J. E. (2004). "I am a puzzle": Adolescence as reflected in self-metaphors. *Canadian Journal of Counselling, 38*(4), 246.

Thomas, G. V. & Jolley, R. P. (1998). Drawing conclusions: A re-examination of empirical and conceptual bases for psychological evaluation of children from their drawings. *British Journal of Clinical Psychology, 37,* 127–139.

Appendix C
Full Methods for Quantitative Analyses (Chapter 4)

Our quantitative analyses in Chap. 4 use data from the Health Behaviour in School-aged Children study. Here we provide background on that data source. We also present an overview of the factor analysis approach that was applied for scale development in each of our three examples of holistic assessment.

The Health Behaviour in School-aged Children (HBSC) Study

Overview

The Health Behaviour in School-aged Children (HBSC) study is conducted in collaboration with the World Health Organization (WHO). The HBSC survey is administered every four years in 44 countries and regions across Europe and North America. The study has been ongoing since 1982, with Canada's participation beginning in 1990. The 2014 survey is Canada's seventh cycle. The survey collects data on health and health-related behaviours of youth aged approximately 11–15 years through a school-based self-report questionnaire. The main purposes of the Canadian HBSC study are to understand youth's health and well-being and to inform education, health policy and health promotion initiatives at provincial/territorial, national, and international levels (Freeman, King, & Pickett, 2015).

Methods

The Sample

The 2014 Canadian HBSC survey targeted a national weighted representative sample. For most provinces, a two-stage cluster sampling approach was used. At the first stage, school jurisdictions were identified and ordered according to key

© The Author(s) 2018
V. Michaelson et al., *Holistic Health in Children: Conceptualization,
Assessment and Potential*, SpringerBriefs in Well-Being and Quality
of Life Research, DOI 10.1007/978-3-319-64831-6

characteristics: language of instruction, public/separate school designation (where applicable), and community size. An ordered list of schools within eligible and consenting jurisdictions was created, and then schools were systematically sampled using a random starting point and fixed sampling interval. Classes had an approximately equal chance of being selected. Administrators at most selected schools were asked to have two classes at each of the selected grades participate. In some of the provinces and territories with larger samples relative to the overall student populations (e.g. Prince Edward Island), all students at selected schools within the targeted grade levels were invited to participate, including all schools and students in the three Territories. Private and special schools, including on-reserve schools, were not included in the study sample to maintain consistency with past survey cycles. These represent <7% of the eligible student population (Freeman, King, & Pickett, 2015).

Response

The 2014 HBSC survey was administered in 377 Canadian schools, and obtained data on a national sample of 29,784 students in grades 6–10. Based upon summary forms provided by teachers of participating classes, the overall student participation rate was estimated at 77%.

Survey Administration. Student questionnaires were administered to school classes, typically by teachers, and were filled out by individual students during one 45–70 minute class. Schools chose to complete the survey either using pen and paper or as a web-based online survey. Almost all of the questions could be answered by checking off a closed-ended response option to the question. There was one version of the questionnaire for Grade 6, 7, and 8 students, and a second longer version for Grade 9 and 10 students.

Ethics and Consent

The researchers were granted ethics clearance for the study by Research Ethics Boards from both Queen's University and PHAC/Health Canada. Consent was passive or active (involving parents), dependent upon the requirements of participating school boards.

Factor Analysis Procedures

All statistical analyses were conducted in SAS Version 9.4 (SAS Institute, Cary, NC). The same general factor analysis procedure was used for each of the holistic measures that were created.

We started by selecting a set of items that were measured in the HBSC and were believed to be theoretically related to the underlying construct. Some items that were highly correlated with other items were excluded. The HBSC dataset was randomly split into two approximately equal halves. Using only one half of the data, we conducted an exploratory factor analysis on all of the items that were preselected. We used the SAS procedure PROC FACTOR with results based upon maximum likelihood estimates. In cases where a one factor solution was desired, we were able to specify a single factor using the nfactor command. Otherwise, we determined the number of factors based on a combination of the eigenvalues (>1), the Scree plot (the elbow), and factor interpretability (Suhr, 2006). In cases where multiple correlated factors were expected, an oblique (promax) rotation was used.

Items were selected for inclusion in the final scale based on their factor loadings (≥ 0.40). If items remaining in the final scale were deemed redundant conceptually, the item with the lower factor loading was dropped. In the case of the overt risk-taking scale, item weights were obtained from the exploratory factor analysis and applied when calculating the summary scores.

Using the second half of the dataset, the above process was repeated. We confirmed model fit using the SAS PROC CALIS procedure. The following statistics are indicative of an acceptable model fit in confirmatory factor analysis: RMSEA of 0.06 or less, SRMR of 0.08 or less, and an AGFI of 0.90 or more (Hu & Bentler, 1999).

The internal consistency (a measure of scale reliability) of the resultant scale was estimated using Cronbach's alpha obtained from the PROC CORR procedure.

The eleven indicators considered for the family systems measure were: (1) relative material wealth, (2) frequency of breakfast consumption, (3) frequency of family meals (breakfast and dinners), (4) number of people in primary home, (5) relative family wealth, (6) ease of communication within family, (7) family support, (8) frequency of screen time on weekdays, (9) family neighbourhood social capital, (10) parental trust and communication, and (11) home climate.

The ten indicators considered for the holistic health measure were: (1) physical activity, (2) sedentary activity (screen time), (3) frequency of breakfast eating, (4) healthy diet, (5) frequency of psychological symptoms, (6) peer support, (7) life satisfaction, (8) student support at school, (9) frequency of somatic symptoms, and (10) spiritual health.

References

Freeman, J., King, M., & Pickett, W. (2015). *Health behaviour in school-aged children (HBSC) in Canada: A focus on relationships*. Ottawa, ON: Public Health Agency of Canada.

Hu, L. T., & Bentler, P. M. (1999). Cutoff criteria for fit indexed in covariance analysis: Conventional criteria versus new alternatives. *Structural equation modeling: A multidisciplinary journal, 6*(1), 1–55.

Suhr, D. D. (2006). *Exploratory or confirmatory factor analysis?* (pp. 1–17). Cary: SAS Institute.